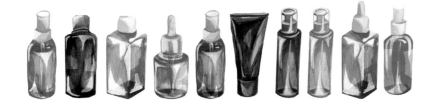

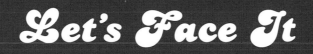

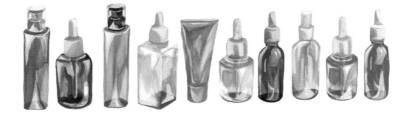

VORACIOUS

Little, Brown and Company
New York Boston London

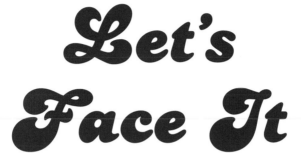

Let's Face It

SECRETS OF A SKINCARE OBSESSIVE

RIO VIERA-NEWTON

Illustrated by Laura Chautin

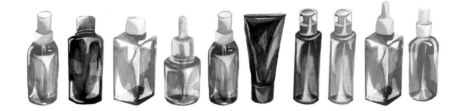

CONTENTS

Let's Face It

INTRODUCTION

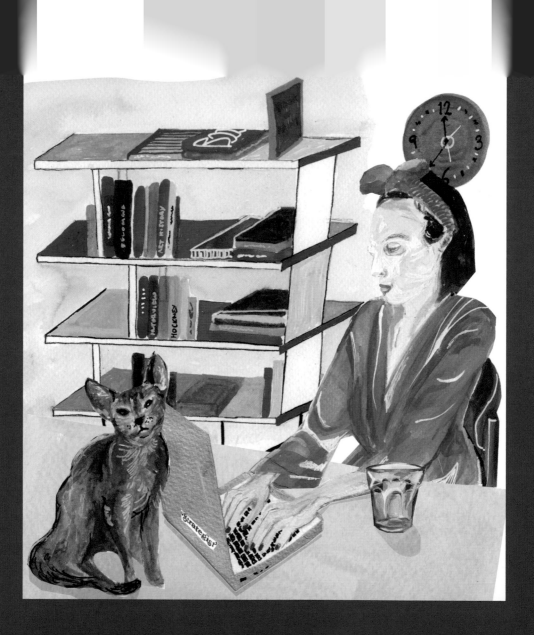

*W*ithout even realizing, we compromise to meet the needs of others every day. You spend a little extra on the dish soap your partner prefers, stay out later than you'd like to attend a friend's party, or walk to a farther coffee shop because your coworker wants to. It's these small acts of accommodation that make us better friends, better colleagues, and better people.

But what do you do each day that's entirely for yourself? For me, it's skincare.

You might recognize my name from my column at *New York* magazine's "The Strategist," where I deconstruct, review, and recommend beauty products every week. On top of sharing my personal experiences with skincare, my articles try to cut through the noise of beautiful packaging, aspirational marketing, and all of the other ways that brands try to convince us we need their products, to find what really works. By obsessively testing skincare products, poring over ingredient lists, and digging deep into each brand's core philosophies, I help people make informed decisions about which products are right for their skin, budget, beliefs, and lifestyle.

Though I now look forward to coming home, tying up my hair, and patting serums and creams onto my skin in front of my bathroom mirror, I wasn't always a bona fide skincare obsessive. For most of my early life, I used whatever products my mom had lying around the house, using a literal bar of soap to wash my face and dabbing on one of her highly fragranced, designer collagen creams afterwards. Whatever personal interest in skincare I had started and ended in the CVS skincare aisle, where I bought products at random based on their pretty packaging or nice-smelling scents.

In my late teenage years, when severe eczema and acne flared up all over my face, I tried everything to get rid of it. I applied prescription-strength acne treatments, which further irritated my skin, and developed bumpy, red patches from overusing intense topical steroids. I used harsh cleansers and scrubs on my already-inflamed skin, hoping I could somehow scrape, burn, and scrub my face clear. But when I went off to college, my hormonal and cystic breakouts seemed to completely disappear. So my ambivalence about what I put on my skin continued. At this point, I refused to wear any makeup, almost as a badge of honor that proved that I was a real adult: I

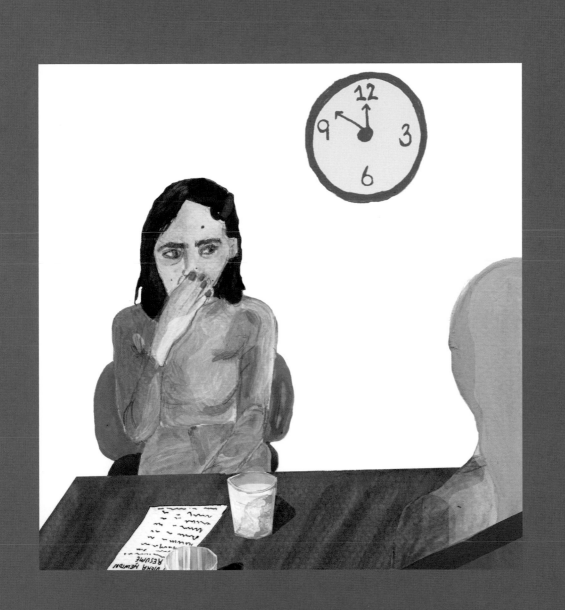

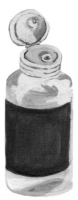

had officially grown up and grown out of my embarrassing teen-age acne.

A few weeks after my graduation from college, out of nowhere, something changed: Each morning I'd wake up with deep, cystic, painful zits that appeared in clusters along my jawline. And my eczema, which I hadn't seen or dealt with in years, re-emerged with a vengeance all across my face. At the time, I was a recent college graduate anxiously job hunting all across New York City. Of course, none of my interviewers judged or even noticed the condition of my skin, but I couldn't help but feel self-conscious. I struggled to make eye contact and covered the inflamed parts of my face with my hand as I spoke. I wasn't confident in my own skin, and this inadvertently affected the ease and comfort in my voice as I spoke. I came across as shy or sheepish, and I just didn't feel like *me.* I would try and wrap up meetings as quickly as possible, desperate to go home, take off my layers of makeup, and pick and prod my skin in the mirror. My obsessive hatred of my skin consumed me, and, un-surprisingly, none of the interviewers I met with called me back.

When I decided to take control of my skin, I barely knew where to start. After many late nights spent sleuthing around the internet, I discovered the Reddit forums r/SkincareAddiction and r/AsianBeauty—online communities that dispensed skincare advice and shared affordable, effective products, many of which catered to sensitive and acne-prone skin. A far cry from the harsh scrubbing cleansers and astringent toners of my teenage years, the products I found nourished and calmed my skin, soothing and hydrating it back to health.

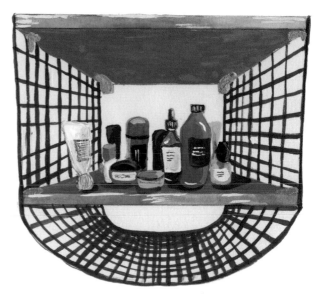

Despite the temptation to dive into an elaborate routine all at once, I knew from my past skincare trials and errors that doing too much often backfired and made it harder to tell what was working. So instead, I slowly integrated each step one by one—first a calming serum, then an exfoliator, then an essence, and so on—until I noticed my skin was less hot and angry and significantly more hydrated. In just a few months, I noticed a huge difference: after years of feeling like my skin had a mind of its own, I finally understood the products and ingredients it craved, and I could avoid the ones it resisted.

My friends also noticed a change—though I think they were mostly grateful

NOT A PROFESSIONAL . JUST CRAZY.

The Google Doc I Send to People Who Ask About My Skin

By Rio Viera-Newton

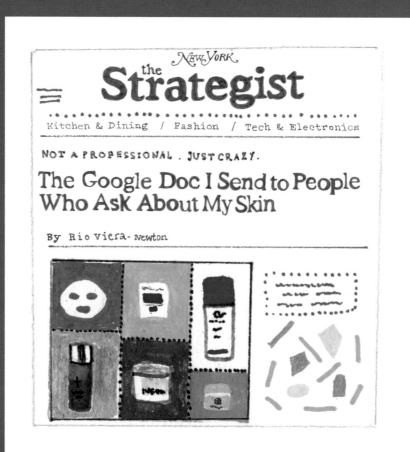

my skin woes were no longer a constant topic of complaint. But when I talked to them about skincare, I realized that they were totally overwhelmed by the sheer amount of information out there: all of the new brands, products, and ingredients were too much for them to keep up with. They asked if I could share some of the things I was using, so I turned my months of research into a simple Google Doc where I casually explained what each product was, how it worked, and how it should be applied to the skin. To my surprise, this Google Doc, originally made for just two close friends, was now being widely shared. People were seeing real results from the products I had recommended, and they were eager to pass along the intel to friends. It got into the hands of other friends, friends of friends, colleagues, and even straight-up strangers, until it finally landed in the inbox of an editor at *New York* magazine's "The Strategist," who asked if she could publish it. The article exploded—it was a "viral" success, selling out my favorite products in a single week—and I was offered a column at "The Strategist" shortly after. I've been writing for them ever since.

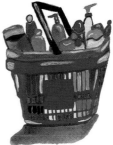

More than three years later, skincare has become one of the fastest-growing industries worldwide, with no signs of slowing down. In the history of cosmetics, there have never been more skincare brands accessible to the public than there are today.

 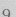

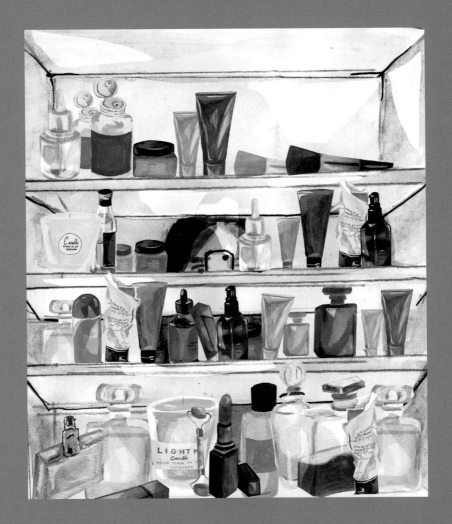

In 2019, the beauty industry was valued at $531 billion. That's a lot of money—and a lot of brands who stand to gain from selling you, the consumer, their product. But it's easier to locate long aisles stacked with beautifully bottled, twenty-dollar night creams than it is to find *impartial* educational material on skincare: lessons that aren't coming straight from a brand with products to sell you. This makes it especially hard to figure out what works for you—what's *actually* good for your skin and what products, ingredients, and steps will help nurture it to a healthy place, as my routine did mine. That's what this book will help you do. Throughout part one, I'll hold your hand as we go over the basics of skincare: what your skin type is, what your skin concerns are, and how we can get a better grasp on what your skin is craving. In part two, I'll talk about ingredients—how they work and which you should look out for or avoid. In part three, we'll deconstruct what all of these skincare products and steps actually do, and in part four, we'll help you build a routine that works for you and your lifestyle.

When you start making skincare a part of your daily life, it can be hard to block out the negative thoughts associated with spending so much time and effort on your appearance. But for me, the effort I put into skincare isn't coming from a narcissistic desire to achieve perfect skin. It's about caring for myself, and making time to do so every day. When I practice my skincare routine, it's one of the only times I feel truly alone with myself and my thoughts. The twenty minutes I spend by myself in the mornings and evenings are invaluable—it's when I'm most able to focus on the day to come and reflect on the day that's passed. I've made some of my most pivotal life decisions while practicing my skincare routine: I made the choice to confront a boss about a raise, pushed myself to leave a toxic relationship, and even mustered up the courage to start writing this book. There's something delightfully introspective about being completely alone, confined to your bathroom, confronting yourself in the mirror (but *not* a magnifying mirror, which no one should have in their home!).

But of course, skincare is not an exclusively cathartic practice. As any acne sufferer knows, healthy skin can completely transform how you feel about yourself. Even today, I'm still very prone to breakouts and clogged pores. But back then, acne had a way of making me feel betrayed by my body: I would frantically think "Why is this happening?" and pile on the foundation or concealer. Nowadays, not only do I feel more equipped to manage flare-ups, I'm easier on myself because I understand my skin and body in ways I hadn't before. Now that my skin and I check in twice a day, every day, I'm more familiar with her patterns and temperaments: She gets angry when I've stayed out late and had one too many cocktails but loves when I get a good night's sleep and glug water all day. A huge lump on my chin usually means my time of the month is about a week away. I

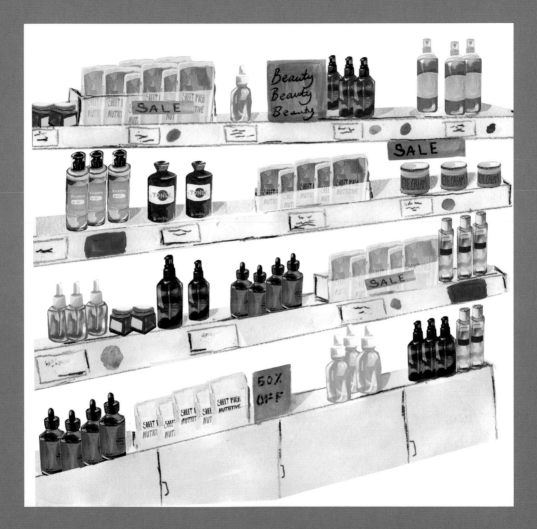

find myself being much more forgiving, if not sympathetic, to my skin's reactive tendencies—I'm less ashamed of my zits because I have a better understanding of why they're there and how to manage them. This is not to say that dramatic breakouts suddenly become less annoying, but spending more time with your skin is really just a way of nurturing a connection with yourself and your body.

A common misconception is that a skincare routine must require an absurd number of time-consuming steps, expensive products, and hot new gadgets. This couldn't be further from the truth. You may be familiar with the idea of the "ten-step routine," created by cosmetic mogul Charlotte Cho to educate consumers on the types of products on the market and a method of layering them. As Charlotte herself has explained, she created the concept of the ten-step routine not to tell people what to use, but to showcase the steps that you can pick and choose from depending on your goals and concerns.

If your skincare routine is so long that you don't feel excited about it or even capable of completing it daily, it's more than okay to slim it down to what's realistic. Skincare requires consistency, so you'll see the best results if you create a routine that you'll diligently stick to and ideally even enjoy practicing. After all, skincare shouldn't feel burdensome, it should be empowering, calming, and therapeutic.

Today, more people than ever are investing time and energy (not to mention money) in skincare. Skincare is now a standard cultural point of reference, brought up in interviews with music giants like Frank Ocean and political leaders like Alexandria Ocasio-Cortez alike. There are now K-beauty-inspired skincare sections in major drugstore chains and thousands of products on the internet that claim to help you "rewind time" or achieve the elusive crystal-clear and perfectly smooth "glass skin." But after reading this book, I want you to walk up to a beauty counter and feel like you know more than any salesperson does. I want you to flip a product around and confidently scan an ingredient list, identifying things you already know your skin does and doesn't respond well to. I want you to know what skincare steps make sense for you: not just for your skin type but also for your daily schedule.

Whether you're a skincare rookie or veteran, this book will help you become your most confident, educated, and aware skincare shopper. I'll go over the ingredients, formulas, and steps you need to know to create your ideal routine, explaining the science behind it all with super-easy-to-digest language, charts, and illustrations. I know it can feel a little intimidating at first (I was petrified before every chemistry test in high school), but I promise you: you've got this.

PART ONE *Let's Get Started*

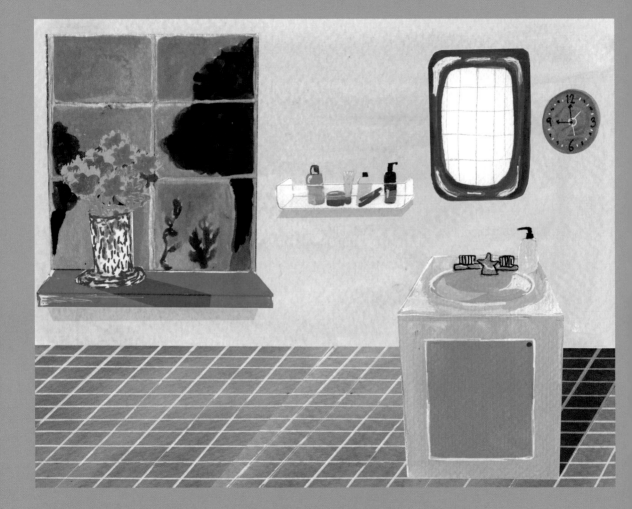

aybe this is the first time you've ventured into the world of skincare. It's possible that you've survived until now with a nondescript moisturizer that you picked up on a whim or a toner your skincare-savvy friend gifted you during a bout of spring cleaning. You've thought about creating a more rigorous skincare routine for yourself—you heard it could help prevent future wrinkles, and, now that you mention it, you've noticed that you break out on your chin from time to time—but you don't know which products are best suited for your skin type or, really, what your skin type even is.

Or perhaps you're a skincare veteran. You stay up-to-date on beauty blogs, watch YouTube reviews, and your medicine cabinet is overflowing with beautiful bottles of all different shapes and sizes. But lately, you've started to feel as though your skin isn't responding to treatments the way it used to. Maybe your skin has begun to feel increasingly sensitive, or drier and duller than usual, and you've noticed that you're more susceptible than ever to breakouts along your jawline. You love skincare, but you want to reassess your products: are they really the best options for your skin type?

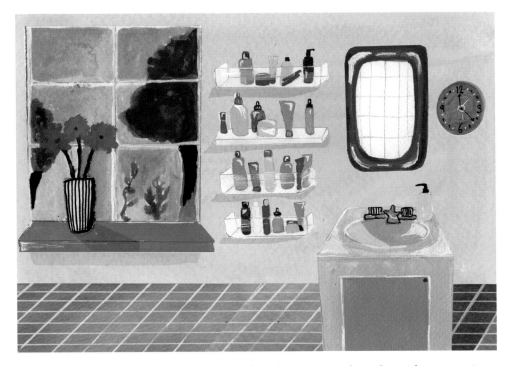

Maybe your skincare routine is right where it needs to be—it's convenient and effective—but you want to deepen your understanding of the science behind the ingredients in your products.

Maybe you're somewhere in the middle.

Regardless of your knowledge of the great big world of beauty, any skincare journey begins with an intimate, one-on-one date with yourself in the mirror. This should be a private experience. Close the door, maybe light a candle for yourself, and take a minute to be and feel alone.

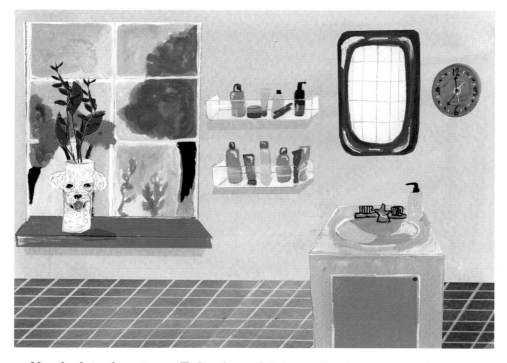

Now look in the mirror. To be clear, this is not the time to consider squeezing that bump you hadn't noticed until now (more on the truly insidious cycle of skin picking later). That's not what we're here to do.

This process isn't about criticizing your skin; it's about working to better understand the fundamental needs of your body. In order to figure out how your skin can look and be its healthiest, we have to figure out where your current routine (or lack thereof) is falling short. Is your skin dehydrated? Is it prone to overproducing oil? Both? Neither? Ultimately, concerns such

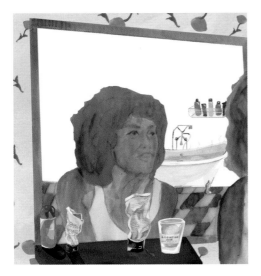

as breakouts or fine lines are merely the by-products of the larger picture of your skin's biological health. So, without judgment, try and imagine describing your skin with detachment, like you would a chair or a flower in a vase: Is it smooth? Is it textured? Is it spotted? Is it blotchy? Is it a bit of all of the above, just in different places?

When analyzing your skin, it's important to take your environment and daily habits into consideration. For example, dark circles, breakouts, and skin dehydration could potentially be linked to things like stress, lack of sleep, or hormones.

The two best times to analyze your skin and determine its type are right when you wake up and in the evening. How your complexion looks and feels when you're completely barefaced in the morning is a helpful way of understanding your skin's baseline. Do you wake up feeling tight and dry? Do you wake up looking a little puffy and blotchy? But your skin is equally telling at the end of the day—you might notice flaky patches where your

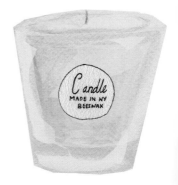

makeup seems to sit on top of your skin, or slippery, shiny spots where oil has collected throughout the day; these are actually helpful indicators of how your skin responds to your daily environment. It's likely you've seen the terms **oily** and **dry** used to define skin types—these terms are ubiquitous in magazines, on the backs of products, and in online reviews, and have been for decades. If you notice a shiny or oily glaze on your skin, that's a sign of over-

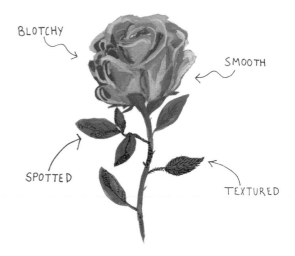

BLOTCHY

SMOOTH

SPOTTED

TEXTURED

production of oil in that area. If you notice rough patches, flakiness, or places where your makeup starts to lift during the day, or if you often wake up with parched, tight-feeling skin, that's a sign of dryness. If an area is neither shiny nor dry—it's mostly just neutral and matte—that's what is commonly referred to as **normal** (though what skin is *ab*normal?).

But, despite what you may have heard, no one skin type is mutually exclusive. It's likely that your skin doesn't necessarily fall under the single category of oily or dry, but is dry in some places and normal or oily in others.

This is what we call **combination skin**. Most people find they have combination skin: when they look in the mirror, they see that they're dry or sensitive in some patches and oily or prone to breakouts in others. Me, I'm oily on my

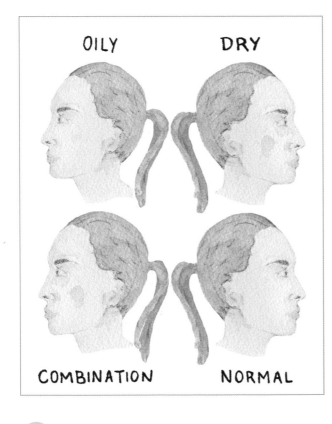

t-zone—the area from the center of my forehead and along the upper brows, all the way down to the tip of my nose and chin— but incredibly, uncomfortably dry around the rest of my face, particularly my cheeks. For me, learning to manage my breakouts has meant, paradoxically, keeping my skin hydrated and soothed, instead of drying it out with harsh astringents. For others, healthy skin might mean controlling and slowing down their skin's over-production of oil with exfoliators, toners, and clay masks. We'll talk more about how to manage skin concerns and treat your particular skin type in the following parts. For now, suffice to say that everybody's body is different, so when curating a routine for yourself, it's important to get to know your skin's quirks. This kind of careful attention in the mirror will pay dividends down the line.

While understanding where your skin lies on the dry/combination/oily/normal scale is a great starting point for interpreting your skin's needs, these terms are clearly not specific enough to describe the full spectrum of skin types. You may look in the mirror and notice, in addition to dryness or oiliness, some redness, spots, scars, or fine lines. Simple terms like *oily, dry,* and *combination* just aren't enough to capture the nuances of how our skin works. It's the largest organ of our body, after all!

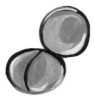

Why Does Oily Skin Get So . . . Oily?

Oily skin occurs when sebaceous glands overproduce sebum, which is the oily and slightly waxy substance in your body that helps to protect and hydrate your skin. But if you've ever hesitated to moisturize your greasiest spots, your

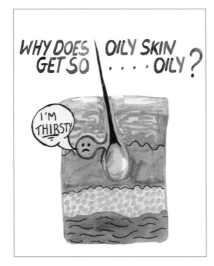

light hand with the moisturizer may have been making things worse: when your skin isn't getting enough hydration, your body overproduces oil to compensate, which can cause the greasy feeling we typically associate with oily skin. Other causes of oily skin can include environmental stressors, such as pollution, climate, or good old genetics. Oily skin tends to collect an excessive amount of dead skin on the surface; this is why people with oily skin tend to be extra susceptible to clogged pores and breakouts. Gentle exfoliation, at least once a week, is a great way for those with oily skin to buff away dead skin and keep breakouts at bay.

Think of your skin like a garden—composed of all different plants and flowers. Yes, there are some general rules of thumb: be patient, don't throw buckets of water and a million different types of fertilizers on it at once and hope for the best, and instead pay close attention to how it changes from week to week and month to month, knowing it might need a bit more hydration in the drier months. But, ultimately, every type of flower in your garden

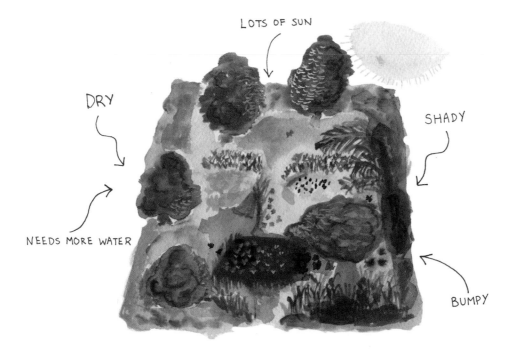

LOTS OF SUN

DRY

SHADY

NEEDS MORE WATER

BUMPY

responds to light, soil, and water in different ways. Some need to be watered daily, others weekly. Some plants thrive in the sun, while others do better in indirect sunlight. The same idea applies to your skin—it's likely that your forehead and cheeks, or nose and jawline, respond to and crave products in different ways. This is not to say that your skin requires a whole pharmacy's worth of different products; it just means that each part of your skin has its own prerequisites and likely interacts with your skincare in unique ways. Are you extra sensitive on your cheeks? Perhaps you don't need to exfoliate there as often as you would, say, your chin, where you notice that you get very oily and congested.

If you suffer from acne, do you notice any kind of pattern? Frequent breakouts along the hairline or outer rim of your face can often be linked to circumstantial changes, such as haircare products with acne-triggering ingredients or even improper cleansing after a long, sweaty workout. Recurring spots from sun damage tend to signify where UV rays are most frequently coming into contact with the skin—historically, the worst sun spots would be concentrated along the center of the face (where the sun would directly hit it), but in recent years, dermatologists have noticed sun spots more frequently appearing on the sides of the face, which many dermatologists believe is linked to blue light rays (high-energy visible light) from cell phones.

How Do I Tell If My Skin Is Sensitive?

Those with sensitive skin can exhibit the qualities of oily, dry, or combination skin types, but they tend to suffer from flare-ups of redness, dehydration, irritation, and, in some cases, even papule breakouts. Typically, these reactions are side effects of environmental stressors like pollution, UV rays, and improper product use.

Determining whether your complexion is oily, dry, normal, or combination will lay down a foundation for understanding your skin. But in order to build a routine that leads to your optimal skin health, we're going to go a little deeper. As someone whose job requires them to stay on top of new launches and innovations, I've tried every product under the sun: masks, ampoules, sleeping packs, toners, exfoliators, cleansers, rollers—you name it—on my face in search of the products that deliver real results. After hundreds of missteps and tons of experimenting, I've found that every product you encounter in a drugstore or a department store beauty counter is designed, or at the very least claims, to address one of the five major pillars of skincare. These pillars are the elements

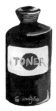

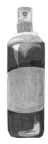

of healthy skin, and when they're in balance, your skin will be calm, nourished, smooth, and bright. These five pillars—**hydrating, healing, plumping, smoothing,** and **illuminating**—go beyond the oily/dry dichotomy to explain the science of skincare and guide you towards products and ingredients best suited for your specific needs.

Most common skin concerns can be addressed through these pillars: textural issues such as acne, as well as bumpy, or rough skin (smoothing); fine lines, wrinkles, or lack of elasticity in the skin (plumping); dryness, dehydration, flaky, or tight skin (hydrating); redness, scabbing, inflammation, and irritation (healing); and dullness, sun spots, and hyperpigmentation (illuminating). These simple, straightforward pillars should be your reliable friends—a guidebook you can refer to any time skincare feels confusing or overwhelming.

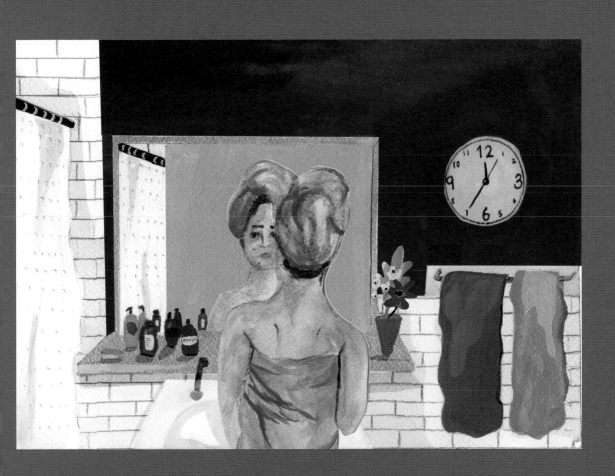

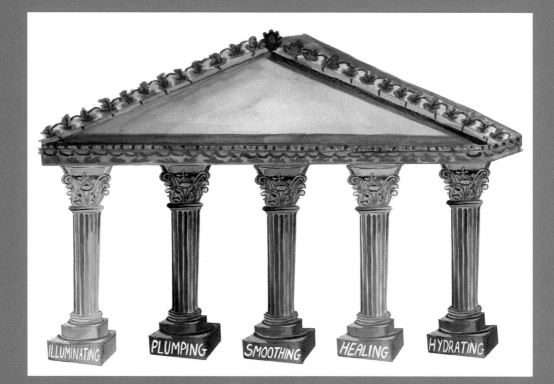

WHICH PILLARS DO
I NEED TO FOCUS ON?

Next, you should analyze your face by touching and feeling it. It's crucial that you always make sure your hands are clean before touching your face, especially if you're prone to breakouts. Wash your hands, then wash them again—pretend you're a doctor about to go into the OR. Looking in the mirror, do you see redness, irritation, breakouts, or flakiness? When you run your (clean!) hands over your face, do you feel bumps or scaly patches? These skin concerns aren't just pesky annoyances; they're actually your key to understanding what your skin craves and/or resists. Most common skin concerns are a sign of an imbalance of one of the pillars of skincare and can be addressed by implementing —or removing —products and ingredients from your routine. Familiarizing yourself with all the pillars, even ones that you might not immediately believe make sense for your skin, is the most effective way to successfully curate a routine that makes the most sense for you. So let's get started!

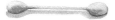

HYDRATING

How Can You Tell If Your Skin Is Dry or Dehydrated?

First and foremost, dehydration is a skin status, while dryness is a skin type. Dryness is due to a general lack of healthy, water-trapping oils called lipids. While skin oils tend to get a bad rap due to their association with greasiness and breakouts, a proper balance of these healthy oils is a pivotal part of maintaining your skin's health. Sebum is rich in lipids, so it helps protect and moisturize the skin. When your skin lacks sebum, it looks and feels dry. If you suffer from dryness, you'll likely notice it on other skin surfaces besides your face: your hands, legs, arms, or even your neck will probably appear flaky, patchy, and parched.

What Is Sebum?

Sebum is the oily substance created by the sebaceous glands that helps keep your body—from your hair to your skin—moisturized. It is made up of triglycerides, fatty acids, and squalene. While balanced sebum levels are essential for skin health, too little or too much can cause dryness or oiliness in the skin.

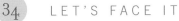

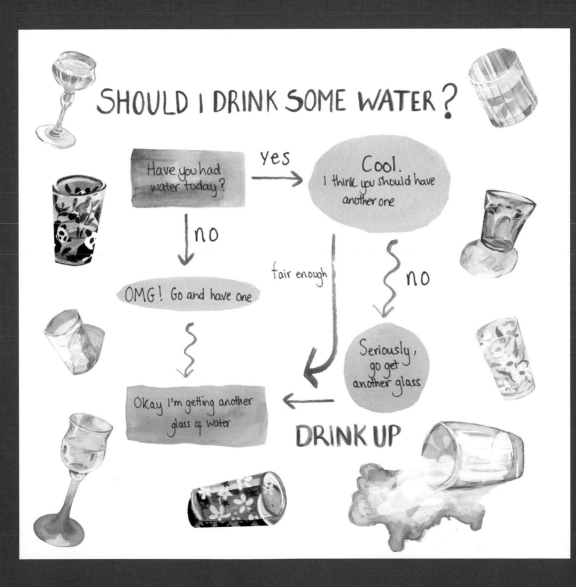

Dehydration, on the other hand, is due to a lack of *water* within the skin and is typically less of a chronic concern. Dehydration is often caused by environmental stressors or incorrectly applied products, so you'll see flare-ups. While drier skin types are more susceptible to dehydration, oily skin can still become dehydrated.

All skin types can benefit from hydration. When dehydrated, oily skin types have a tendency to overproduce oil, which can often cause breakouts. This can be experienced not just during drier climate conditions (like winter months), but also when using a drying skincare regimen to try and combat skin oiliness. Paradoxically, integrating a lightweight, gel-based moisturizer into your routine during acne flare-ups and avoiding drying or irritating skincare products can help rebalance the skin and prevent acne.

Dry skin types, however, can always benefit from hydration.

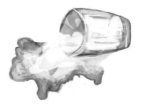

Common Causes of Dehydration

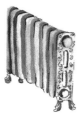

Intense air-conditioning or heating systems in your home or office

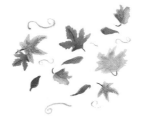

Cold and/or windy weather

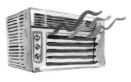

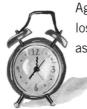

Aging (Your skin loses moisture as you age.)

Improper skincare (This usually means over-exfoliating or ingredients that are too harsh for you.)

Hot showers or baths (I know they're lovely, but they actually are stripping on the skin!)

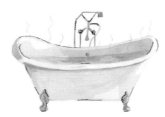

HEALING

Healing addresses any kind of skin irritation, whether it be scabs, redness, inflammation, scaliness, or even old breakouts (anything from an old whitehead to a cyst on its way out). Healing ingredients deeply soothe and nurture the skin and can rehabilitate any kind of damage due to environmental stressors (the sun, pollution, allergic reactions) or chemical reactions (from over-exfoliating or other cosmetic damage). They can have rejuvenating properties that increase cell turnover to promote faster wound healing, as well as calming and anti-inflammatory properties.

Cell Turnover

Cell turnover refers to the shedding of old, dead skin cells and the subsequent replacement with fresh, new, young cells. A healthy amount of cell shedding is essential both on the very surface of the skin and deep in the pores. Certain ingredients help promote the process of cell turnover by stimulating the removal of old skin cells and then accelerating the emergence of new cells.

Acid exfoliators, such as AHAs, BHAs, and PHAs (more on those later), also help remove dead skin cells from the surface of the skin and in the pores, but can be quite abrasive and stripping when used too frequently. Healing ingredients, on the other hand, can promote cell turnover while also hydrating and soothing the skin.

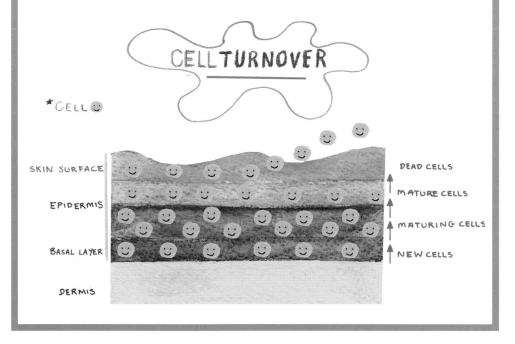

PLUMPING

Some people may observe fine lines and wrinkles around the eyes, around the mouth (smile lines), or on the forehead. These are caused by a variety of factors, the most common of which are dehydration and aging. As we age, our natural levels of hyaluronic acid (which traps water in the dermis, the top layer of skin), collagen, and elastin decrease, causing wrinkles, sagging skin, and fine lines. If vitality, elasticity, and/or bouncy skin are goals of yours, plumping products dive deep into your skin, nourishing and invigorating your body's natural hyaluronic acid–, collagen- and elastin-building processes.

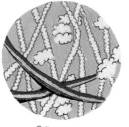 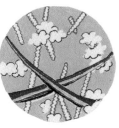 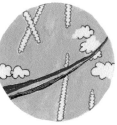

35 YEARS   45 YEARS   55 YEARS

HYALURONIC ACID
COLLAGEN
ELASTIN

SMOOTHING

If rough patches, consistent breakouts, or clogged pores are an issue for you, incorporating smoothing ingredients and products can help refine, resurface, and even out a bumpy complexion. Some active ingredients in smoothing products, which include chemical exfoliators and retinoids, tend to be some of the most intense on the market, so being mindful of where and how often you apply them, and only treating areas that really need help, is important for ensuring that your skin remains balanced and healthy without being stripped. We'll talk more about how to use these products responsibly later. For now, just know to start slow and take everything one step at a time: there's no need to panic-buy a million different products.

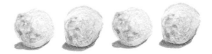

ILLUMINATING

While smoothing ingredients can help target and treat the causes of acne, illuminating is the pillar to consider when your zits are on their way out. Whether you're hoping to tackle post-inflammatory hyperpigmentation or erythema left behind by breakouts, hormonal pigmentation (also known as melasma), or sun spots, products that incorporate illuminating ingredients will help even out your complexion and deliver an allover glow to the skin.

But not only those who suffer from acne can reap the benefits of these ingredients. Because of illuminating's wide benefits, it's kind of a catchall for people of most ages and skin types: someone in their early twenties who suffers from acne scarring, as well as someone in their sixties who's looking to improve dull, tired skin can see results from incorporating more illuminating products into their routine.

ACNE

Acne sufferers reading this book may wonder how I can talk about skincare without confronting the elephant in the room: acne. According to the American Academy of Dermatology, acne is the most common skin condition in the United States, affecting up to 50 million Americans annually. Despite it being one of the most talked about and diagnosed skin concerns, it's not the be-all and end-all of skin health. In fact, it's just one facet of your skin's overall condition. If you suffer from consistent bumps or breakouts 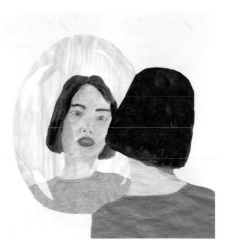 (whether that be a patch of little closed bumps, whiteheads, or deep and cystic zits), skin-smoothing products can be incredibly helpful tools to help resurface your complexion and manage the root of these flare-ups. However, learning how to properly integrate these intensive treatments into your regimen, without stripping or irritating the skin, can be a finicky process. If you're acne prone as well as sensitive, like I am, it's important that you balance the harshness of smoothing skincare products with ingredients that fall under

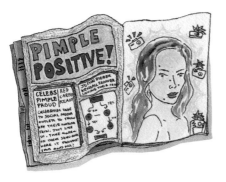

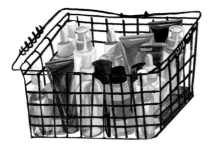

the healing and hydrating pillars. That way, your skin won't get stripped of its natural moisture and appear even more red and irritated. However, if your skin is on the oilier side and you suffer from breakouts, a routine that uses smoothing products more frequently may be more suitable for you. It's all about trying things out—building up or cutting back on how often you use certain products—until your skin looks its best, without redness, irritation, flakiness, or significantly more breakouts.

As I sit here and preach the importance of embracing your skin—nurturing it towards a healthy state rather than battering it with harsh products—I'm fully aware that those of you who suffer from acne may be thinking "Sure, if you have perfect skin." I know, because I've been through the psychological burden of battling long-term, fluctuating cystic and hormonal acne. Here's what I wish I knew back then: nowadays, there are more cases of adult hormonal acne than there have ever been reported. You are not alone. And because of this widespread skin condition, acne-prone skin is more frequently being used as an example of the norm. Everyone breaks out, and that's finally being represented. We are no longer subject to the illusion that everyone but us has perfect skin. Celebrities like Saoirse Ronan, Lorde, and even Justin Bieber are comfortable talking about their journeys with acne in interviews and on Instagram (zit cream and all!). And beauty giants like *Teen Vogue* are willing to do unretouched editorial shoots with real skin, and often that means no makeup at all. We are getting to a place where we're finally willing to admit that acne isn't so unusual—it's a part of being human.

But on a cosmetic level, what this means is more investment in understanding, accepting, and caring for acne-prone skin. Historically, those with acne were told by magazines and brands alike that they had to use harsh and astringent face washes and topical creams to clear up breakouts. Nowadays, more companies use sensitivity as the archetype for their typical acne-prone consumer.

While I believe that acceptance of one's skin is essential, there is absolutely no harm in understanding the science behind your skin and the products that can help. Deconstructing the anatomy of acne—how it's triggered and soothed—can allow you to make more intuitive, informed decisions when it comes to your skincare.

What Is Acne, Anyway?

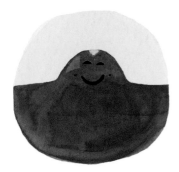

Acne is a skin condition that occurs when a pore is clogged, creating inflamed, often painful bumps on the skin. Different types of clogs create different forms of acne. Consistent acne sufferers can see great results from regulated uses of ingredients that fall under the smoothing pillar, which can help exfoliate dead skin cells and control the excess oil production that triggers acne. Healing ingredients can also work in conjunction with these smoothing treatments to soothe and calm irritation or redness caused by breakouts and even speed up their recovery time.

Hormonal acne is not a type of blemish, but a cause of acne. Hormonal acne is usually set off by a change in your body's hormone levels; this can be triggered by anything from your time of the month to your immune system to stress. Since hormonal acne is caused by what is going on internally, as opposed to external triggers (like a bad product), it's likely that it will be more persistent and recur in the same places over and over again. For people who menstruate, dermatologists will sometimes encourage balancing out your hormones with birth control pills (in consultation with an ob-gyn). Others, including some dermatologists, believe that drinking lots of water can help prevent excess oil production, which can possibly contribute to hormonal acne.

Whiteheads are the product of a pore getting clogged with dead skin, bacteria, and oils. The pore closes, all that gunk gets trapped, and it shows up as a little white bump above the surface of your skin. These are kind of like baby zits—they don't usually swell or redden the way a pustule would. Honestly, you might not even notice them until you're in harsh lighting or up close. If you have just a few, they will typically go away on their own in the shower, or, with a little spot treatment, they should disappear in a few days.

Pustules are a meaner version of the above. They're what you might think of as the most conventional kind of pimple. As in, if you had to draw a zit from memory, odds are it would probably look like this. Unlike whiteheads, pustules are inflamed and can be painful. They occur when a blackhead or whitehead gets so irritated that its cellular membrane breaks, and the swelling and inflammation form a larger, more aggressive pimple. But again, these are relatively easy to treat—with smoothing products or treatments—as long as you don't worsen the area by picking and prodding.

Blackheads are another kind of blemish you're likely familiar with. We all

When Should You Pop a Pimple?

Popping—sometimes called **extraction**—is exactly as it sounds: bursting a pimple and squeezing out the dead cell debris or pus trapped in the pore. While many people believe that popping zits can speed up the recovery time of a pimple, a premature extraction can actually damage the skin, creating a post-inflammatory hyperpigmentation or erythema mark that can last for weeks, months, or even years. My best advice is, please don't pop your zit. But if you absolutely can't resist, it should be popped only when pus is visible. When pus appears, you should wrap your two index fingers in toilet paper and gently squeeze. I have a three-strike rule: if nothing comes out in three tries, I stop. If you need to be extremely aggressive, it means the pimple isn't ready. Squeezing a pimple before its time can lead to excessive scarring and longer healing times.

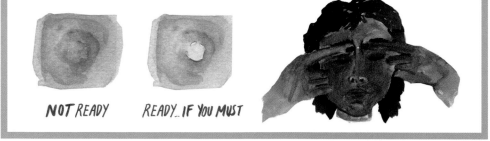

NOT READY   READY... IF YOU MUST

have them. Like whiteheads, they're little plugs of oils, sebum, and bacteria that clog the surface of your skin. Blackheads are actually a result of when that pore bursts open, oxidizing the oil and creating a little, dark-colored lump or dot. Blackheads are best treated during facial sessions; a certified esthetician with appropriate and safe extraction and steaming tools can remove the bacteria and pus in a nondamaging way. At-home blackhead extractions, when done incorrectly, can create a blemish bigger than the tiny little blackhead was in the first place. And I should say this: those blackhead pore strips we've all seen since the nineties are pretty much just as bad as picking at your skin. They're often filled with stripping astringents and alcohols, not to mention they're basically just ripping natural oils out of your skin. When it comes to steady prevention of blackheads, consistent use of a retinoid is one of the most effective things you can do. I'll talk a lot about the benefits and science of retinoids later.

Papules are little tiny bumps on your skin. While all zits are better left undisturbed, these are the ones you absolutely should not touch or mess with. These tiny red bumps can be found alone or in clusters, and they have nothing in them—no whitehead or blackhead to be extracted or squeezed out. Much to the chagrin of poppers everywhere, trying to pinch these can only hurt, not help, and can cause redness or permanent scarring. Papules can oftentimes

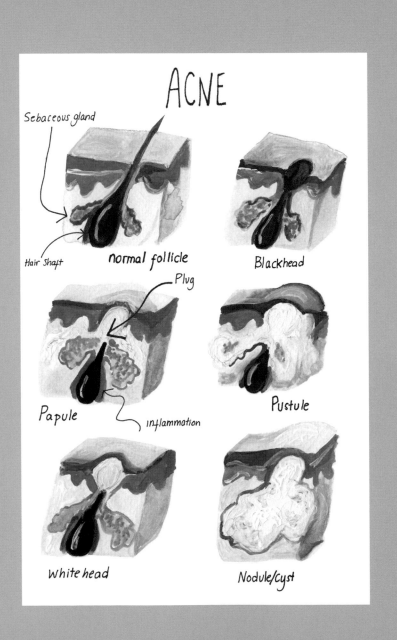

be a result of skin conditions such as eczema or psoriasis. When you get a bug bite, that inflammation is also considered a papule. Milia—those tiny, annoying white bumps that can sprout up in groups—are also papules. In most cases, papules are more of an eyesore than they are painful, but do me a favor and leave your papules alone. If you are suffering from persistent papules, visiting a dermatologist for a prescription for Retin-A (a type of retinoid) or an antibiotic treatment is your best option.

Cysts are nestled deep in the skin and filled with pus—this makes them soft, yet painful to touch. Acne cysts are filled with pus and are a result of an infection deep in the skin. Acne cysts pop up when the pus in blackheads and whiteheads "spills" into other areas of the skin. The skin responds by creating more pus, which further triggers inflammation. Cysts can be treated with smoothing treatments, such as benzoyl peroxide (which can help decrease swelling and exfoliate dead skin), or, in severe cases, a dermatologist can drain the cyst or reduce its size with a cortisone injection. I would only recommend a cortisone injection if you have had a persistent cyst that hasn't gone away for months.

Nodules are the most severe kind of acne. They are solid-feeling lumps that, like cystic acne, develop due to an infection deep in the skin. They are solid lumps under the skin that develop from infected and irritated papules and pustules, growing angrier, bigger, and deeper into the skin. Unlike cysts, nodules are quite hard and feel like rocks underneath the top layer of skin. If you suffer from nodules, you should consult a dermatologist—nodules can cause severe scarring and damage to the skin and should absolutely not be messed with.

Seeing a Dermatologist

If you suffer from recurring or consistent skin concerns such as acne, eczema, psoriasis, or severe scarring, you should consider getting the opinion of a dermatologist before creating an at-home routine. A dermatologist can help you understand what products or ingredients are most suitable for your exact skin condition and avoid the ingredients that may trigger flare-ups. While some patients prefer to see their dermatologist more regularly, others only see them once every few years to check in. Researching doctors is important when looking for one that's best for your skin's needs. While all dermatologists have a wealth of knowledge when it comes to skin, you may want to look for a dermatologist who specializes in your specific skin concern to receive more specialized attention.

Grades of Acne

When visiting a dermatologist, they'll often reference this grading system to measure the intensity, location, and severity of blemishes. Familiarizing yourself with this language may help you better communicate your history or current skin status to your doctor.

Grade 1—Mild. Primarily blackheads and whiteheads.

Grade 2—Moderate. Papules and pustules, primarily on the face.

Grade 3—Moderate to severe. A combination of papules and pustules, with the possibility of cysts and nodules. Not limited to the face (may affect the back and chest).

Grade 4—Severe. A large number of painful pustules, papules, and nodules.

All grades can benefit from a doctor visit, but grades 3 and 4 can see the best results if and when they are prescribed oral or topical remedies by a dermatologist.

ACNE SCARS

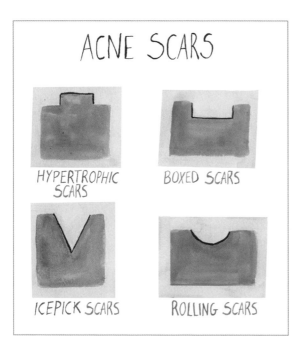

ACNE SCARS

HYPERTROPHIC SCARS

BOXED SCARS

ICEPICK SCARS

ROLLING SCARS

If acne is an issue for you, it's likely that scarring is as well. When a swollen, inflamed acne lesion flattens out—whether it be through extraction or healing of its own accord—a scar or mark is typically left behind. There are varying degrees of acne scars: some can appear as just a slight shadow, while others are the product of deeper, more intense cystic pimples and can have a lasting effect on the texture and pigment of the skin. There are a few different kinds of scarring that can occur on the skin: pigmentation damage (known as post-inflammatory hyperpigmentation or post-inflammatory erythema), raised lumps (known as hypertrophic or keloid scars), or indents (known as atrophic scarring). Your body has a natural healing process for combating scarring, but skincare products and treatments can work with your body's natural cycles to help promote and stimulate a more rapid recovery and protect it from further damage. Understanding the type of scar you're dealing with will help guide you towards the treatments that may be helpful.

Post-inflammatory Hyperpigmentation

Post-inflammatory hyperpigmentation (PIH) develops when a wound, rash, pimple, or other trauma causes skin inflammation. As the skin heals, it produces too much melanin (the substance that gives skin its color), leaving a bruise-like mark behind. Illuminating skincare ingredients are vital to helping lift marks left behind due to PIH.

Post-inflammatory Erythema

Unlike PIH, **post-inflammatory erythema** (PIE) is caused by capillary issues or by an influx of inflammation caused by white blood cells (giving an area increased blood pooling and therefore some redness), rather than an overproduction of melanin. This is why PIE appears pinker than PIH. If you put pressure on the area and the color seems to temporarily fade, that means it is post-inflammatory erythema rather than hyperpigmentation. Like PIH, it can be treated with ingredients that fall under the illuminating pillar.

Unlike PIE and PIH, the kinds of acne scars I'm about to list can't be treated with skincare alone. While illuminating treatments may reduce any pigmentation issues around the area, you'll need to consult a dermatologist about treating their appearance.

Ice-Pick Scars

Ice-pick scars are deep linear or v-shaped scars that occur when an infected cyst manages to reach the surface of the skin. The tissue demolished during this process then leaves behind a long, linear scar.

Rolling Scars

This type of scar has a kind of wavy appearance to it and isn't particularly defined. Rolling scars form when the deeper layers of the skin and the surface of the skin develop a fibrous tissue between them, due to acne wounds.

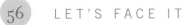

Boxcar Scars

These scars can look craggy, almost like craters in the skin. They're caused when an inflammatory breakout erodes the skin's natural collagen, producing a depression in the skin. Boxcar scars can be mild to severe, depending on how much tissue was lost and/or damaged.

Keloid Scars

Keloid scars are raised overgrowths of scar tissue that occur after the skin is damaged by cystic or nodular acne. The most effective way to get rid of acne keloids is with cryosurgery, which uses liquid nitrogen to freeze off the scarring.

· · ·

Now that you have some idea which pillars of skincare make the most sense for your skin type, we'll dive deep into the ingredients that will help. Admittedly, this might involve interpreting some names of chemicals that you might have found intimidating before—and reading the fine print to figure out just what the heck each product is actually doing—but it's also where the fun starts.

PART TWO

What's Inside Your Products?

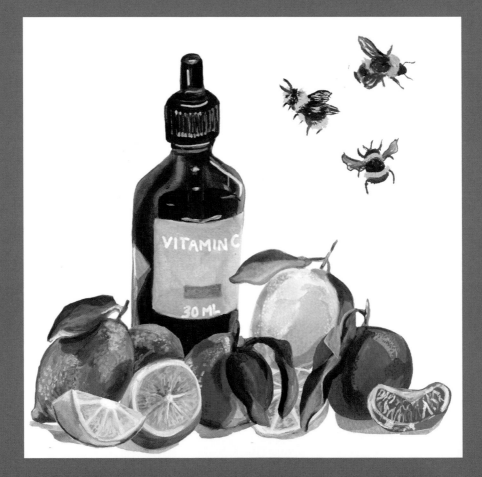

*I*n the previous part, we talked about how your complexion can be better understood through the prism of the five pillars of skincare: hydrating, healing, plumping, smoothing, and illuminating. But what exactly should you look out for when you're shopping for skincare products? With our endless access to cosmetics, it's easy to fall victim to the constant media circus promoting "buzzy" products—new launches, must-have toners, and holy-grail serums endorsed by celebrities, influencers, and at some point maybe even me! But just because *they* love a product, it doesn't mean it's right for you. Armed with some basic knowledge about what different ingredients in skincare accomplish—and with a sense of which ingredients you should avoid—you can cut through the noise of advertising and influencers to figure out what products can actually benefit your skin type. In this part, we're going to familiarize ourselves with ingredient lists, taking apart the scientific gibberish on the labels of your favorite products to figure out what they're actually doing on your skin.

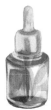

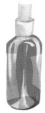

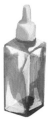

Typically, the only information we have easy access to when shopping is curated by the brands themselves, with pseudo-educational descriptions and instructions that more often than not insist you have to purchase other products from the brand for best results. Buzzwords like *clean* and *natural*, which are all over labels, aren't even official terms regulated by the FDA—they're just marketing tools used to create a sense of safety.

If you're cautious about the ingredients in your cosmetics—if, for example, you want to avoid sensitizing or stripping products, or if you're prone to acne, it can be tough to trust brands at face value. The truth is, they'll always lean towards language that's persuasive to as many people as possible. No brand wants you to pick up their product and think it's not suitable for you.

The only way to figure out what a product really contains and what those contents really do is to read the ingredient list. And, believe me, I know that's no easy feat! My first attempt at reading the ingredient list on the back of a product felt a bit like trying to translate another language—a medical dialect with a few familiar words like *honeysuckle* or *willow bark* floating in a sea of unpronounceable chemicals. In this part, I want to give

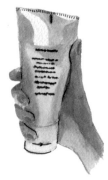

you the tools not just to know what these chemical words mean, but also to understand what the ingredients actually do for your skin. You'll be able to avoid ingredients that don't work for you, and ensure that a product promising "lifted and firm skin" actually has ingredients that fight fine lines or prevent premature aging.

INGREDIENT LISTS AT A GLANCE

Ingredients are listed in descending order by weight, from highest to lowest concentration (with the exception of anything concentrated below 1 percent). This means that the first line of an ingredient list, namely the first five to six ingredients, will tell you a whole lot about both the product and the brand who makes it. For example, if a cream is marketed as a "nourishing propolis cream," but propolis is one of the last ingredients listed, you certainly have a right to be skeptical. However, all ingredients work and deliver effective results at different concentrations, so just because a star ingredient isn't in the first line, it doesn't necessarily mean the product is bad. Having said that, if you see ingredients you *don't* like in the first line of the list (more on what you might want to avoid shortly), you should steer clear of the product.

Before we get into becoming an empowered skincare consumer, let's talk about the products you already own. Be honest: do you have a moisturizer or cleanser that's been sitting in your medicine cabinet for months or maybe even years? Let's figure out whether it's expired or still good to go. The easiest products to decipher are the ones that are classified as over the counter (OTC) by the FDA, which include sunscreens and many acne products that contain active ingredients like salicylic acid or benzoyl peroxide at high concentrations. OTC products have a "Drug Facts" box on the back, where you can find the expiration date. If the product is also registered and sold in Europe, it will have a small illustration of a jar with a number in the middle showing how long the product is safe to use after opening. It's usually somewhere between six and twelve months.

If you see neither of these options, it can be helpful to write the date of opening in Sharpie on the bottle—if it's been less than a year, it's usually still good

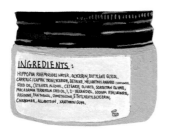

to use. However, how you've maintained the product can also affect its life span: if a product has been sitting by a window in direct sunlight, in a stuffy, hot space, or with the cap not properly screwed on, it's likely to expire quicker than a product in an airtight container in a cool, dark space. Also, if the consistency of the formula doesn't look the same as it did when you first opened it (it's runnier, thicker, or significantly more separated), or if it has a different color or smell, it's likely expired.

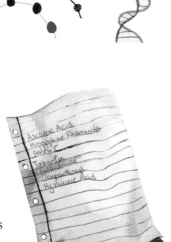

All skincare ingredients are chemicals—even water!—and each chemical, no matter how large or small the percentage included, will elicit a response from your skin. This is why understanding the basic science behind how each ingredient interacts with one another, as well as with your skin, is essential for selecting the best skincare for you. Of course, there are hundreds and thousands of ingredients in the world, so not even close to every one will be discussed in this book. But I've created a list of some of my favorites, as well as some of the most popular in skincare right now, so you can better understand the products you might either already own or plan to buy. These ingredients make up my skincare varsity team. But if you encounter ingredients that don't come up in this book while you're out in the wild, a quick Google Scholar search should at least point you in the direction of an article or medical journal that will help explain what its purpose is in your product.

Take a second and check the ingredients listed on your favorite products. If you feel totally overwhelmed by the sheer number of ingredients, don't fret.

This book is your new best friend. Just as it was in my high school chemistry classes, taking notes was crucial to bettering my understanding of ingredient lists. That way, it wasn't necessary for me to repeatedly look up a specific chemical word. I added to a list on my phone every time I researched an ingredient—noting its scientific name, what it allegedly does, and whether or not it worked for me—and began to compile a glossary to guide me. This list grew and grew, evolving into a working document that I could whip out whenever I was shopping to easily explain what I was looking at. It also allowed me to see how many different words there are for one single ingredient. Suddenly, the ingredient lists didn't seem so insanely daunting.

Skincare ingredients can often have a few different results on your skin, some you might not even expect or immediately notice. Remember earlier, when you looked in the mirror and examined where your skin might need additional love? Each of the pillars of skincare have ingredients that address them, helping to replenish that aspect of your skin. The active ingredients in most skincare products fall under one of the pillars: hydrating, illuminating, plumping, healing, and smoothing. But most ingredients don't fall exclusively in one category—for example, an ingredient that falls under the healing pillar can also have some illuminating and smoothing benefits—so we'll use handy charts to characterize the many ways in which an ingredient acts on your skin.

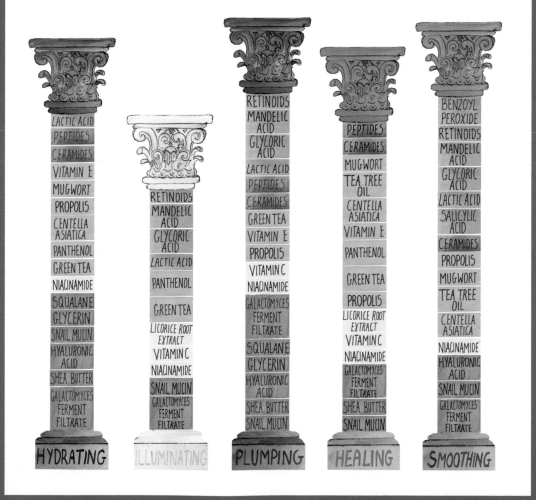

THE FIVE PILLARS OF SKINCARE

HYDRATING
- LACTIC ACID
- PEPTIDES
- CERAMIDES
- VITAMIN E
- MUGWORT
- PROPOLIS
- CENTELLA ASIATICA
- PANTHENOL
- GREEN TEA
- NIACINAMIDE
- SQUALANE
- GLYCERIN
- SNAIL MUCIN
- HYALURONIC ACID
- SHEA BUTTER
- GALACTOMYCES FERMENT FILTRATE

ILLUMINATING
- RETINOIDS
- MANDELIC ACID
- GLYCORIC ACID
- LACTIC ACID
- PANTHENOL
- GREEN TEA
- LICORICE ROOT EXTRACT
- VITAMIN C
- NIACINAMIDE
- SNAIL MUCIN
- GALACTOMYCES FERMENT FILTRATE

PLUMPING
- RETINOIDS
- MANDELIC ACID
- GLYCORIC ACID
- LACTIC ACID
- PEPTIDES
- CERAMIDES
- GREEN TEA
- VITAMIN E
- PROPOLIS
- VITAMIN C
- NIACINAMIDE
- GALACTOMYCES FERMENT FILTRATE
- SQUALANE
- GLYCERIN
- HYALURONIC ACID
- SHEA BUTTER
- SNAIL MUCIN

HEALING
- PEPTIDES
- CERAMIDES
- MUGWORT
- TEA TREE OIL
- CENTELLA ASIATICA
- VITAMIN E
- PANTHENOL
- GREEN TEA
- PROPOLIS
- LICORICE ROOT EXTRACT
- VITAMIN C
- NIACINAMIDE
- GALACTOMYCES FERMENT FILTRATE
- SHEA BUTTER
- SNAIL MUCIN

SMOOTHING
- BENZOYL PEROXIDE
- RETINOIDS
- MANDELIC ACID
- GLYCORIC ACID
- LACTIC ACID
- SALICYLIC ACID
- CERAMIDES
- PROPOLIS
- MUGWORT
- TEA TREE OIL
- CENTELLA ASIATICA
- NIACINAMIDE
- HYALURONIC ACID
- SNAIL MUCIN
- GALACTOMYCES FERMENT FILTRATE

Active vs. Inactive Ingredients

On an ingredient list (primarily for sunscreens and acne products), when you see "Active Ingredients" listed on the back, it means that the key ingredients in the product's formula have been approved by the FDA to treat a specific condition. For example, in products that claim to treat acne, salicylic acid is a common active ingredient.

However, "active ingredients" is also an unofficial term used in skincare to describe the workhorse ingredients in products; it is a way of explaining which ingredients in a formula actually deliver the proposed results. Inactive ingredients do serve a purpose as well: they usually act as hydrating cushions or stabilizers to the active ingredient.

Now let's talk about the ingredients that address the pillars of skincare that are of particular concern to you. But don't rush out and start shopping just yet. In the next part, we'll talk about the wild world of products: how to shop for them and use them and what all those serums and ampoules actually do.

HYDRATING

Hydration is key if your skin often feels rough or dry to the touch or if you spot dry or flaky bits on your skin throughout the day. If you're used to coming home with your makeup peeling or scaling, that's a telltale sign that your routine should address skin dryness or dehydration. But even if you're not prone to dryness, every routine should include hydrating ingredients. Moisture is the foundation of skin health—a proper balance of hydration is essential for achieving a healthy lipid barrier and radiant skin. Here are the ingredients you should seek out in your products:

Shea Butter

Also falls under **Healing** and **Plumping**
Can also be found in ingredient lists as
  · *Butyrospermum parkii*

Shea butter is a fatty acid- and vitamin-rich emollient that's used to help moisturize, replenish, and smooth dry skin. Shea butter also works as an occlusive, or moisture blocker, which is why it's typically found in moisturizers—it helps lock hydration into the skin by creating a protective seal on the surface, preventing it from evaporating into the atmosphere. Because of this, shea butter also has some healing properties. Most skin types can use shea butter, though its richness may be an issue for those with particularly oily skin.

What Is an Emollient?

Emollients are ingredients that help smooth, hydrate, and soften the skin to combat dryness or scaliness. Emollients can either work as humectants, which attract water to the surface of the skin, or as occlusives, which help keep water from evaporating. Emollients are great for drier skin types, but those with oily and acne-prone skin might find formulas with emollients in them to be overly conditioning.

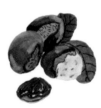

What Is an Occlusive?

Occlusives work to create a seal over the skin that helps trap moisture in the dermis and protect the surface of the skin. Occlusive agents are often found in rich, nourishing moisturizers. The word *occlusive* can also be used to describe products like sheet masks that physically put a barrier between the skin and its environment.

Galactomyces Ferment Filtrate

Also falls under **Illuminating, Plumping, Healing, and Smoothing**

Galactomyces ferment filtrate (say that five times fast) is a yeast-derived ingredient popular in Korean and Japanese cosmetics. It's actually a by-product of the process of fermenting sake, or rice wine. Though fermented ingredients have only recently become more common in cosmetics, some studies have suggested that fermentation naturally boosts the antioxidant, vitamin, and peptide count in a substance, and, when applied topically, these ingredients help restore the skin's natural moisture barrier and prevent water loss. There's also some research that shows that galactomyces ferment filtrate's high nutrient count can help smooth textural issues, diminish hyperpigmentation, and control sebum and acne.

Hyaluronic Acid

Also falls under **Plumping** *and* **Smoothing**
Can also be found in ingredient lists as

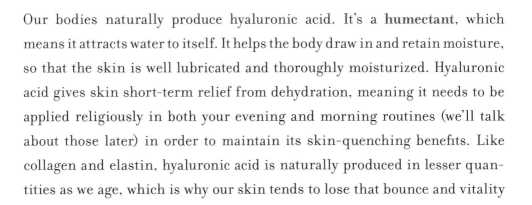

- *Sodium hyaluronate (a salt derivative of hyaluronic acid that purportedly penetrates deeper and quicker into the skin)*

Our bodies naturally produce hyaluronic acid. It's a **humectant**, which means it attracts water to itself. It helps the body draw in and retain moisture, so that the skin is well lubricated and thoroughly moisturized. Hyaluronic acid gives skin short-term relief from dehydration, meaning it needs to be applied religiously in both your evening and morning routines (we'll talk about those later) in order to maintain its skin-quenching benefits. Like collagen and elastin, hyaluronic acid is naturally produced in lesser quantities as we age, which is why our skin tends to lose that bounce and vitality as we grow older. This is why applying hyaluronic acid topically can provide wonderful plumping and skin-smoothing benefits as well as moisturizing ones.

Tip

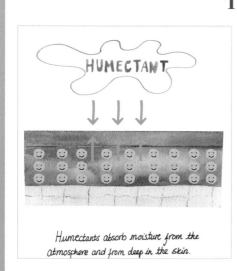

Humectants absorb moisture from the atmosphere and from deep in the skin.

Since hyaluronic acid is a humectant, your skin needs to be wet when you're applying an HA-based product. You can either splash your skin with water or apply your HA-based product after a water-based product, like an essence or serum, in order to achieve the skin-quenching benefits of hyaluronic acid.

Glycerin

Also falls under **Plumping**

Can also be found in ingredient lists as

- *Glyceryl behenate*
- *Batyl alcohol*

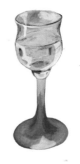

Like hyaluronic acid, glycerin is a humectant, which means it attracts water. It pulls water from deeper layers of the skin into the outer layer so that the skin looks and feels more moisturized. If it's humid out, it will even draw in moisture from the air. This additional moisture gives the skin a nourished, quenched, and plumping effect.

People often ask what the difference is between hyaluronic acid and glycerin, as they are both effective, commonly used humectants in skincare. The biggest difference between the two on a chemical level is in how they distribute moisture throughout your skin. As an ingredient, hyaluronic acid is a larger molecule, so it sits on top of the skin, creating a cushion of moisture on the upper epidermis. Glycerin, on the other hand, is (in general) a smaller molecule, so it can penetrate deep down into the skin to pull water towards the surface, as well as pull moisture from the atmosphere. Another, arguably important distinction between hyaluronic acid and glycerin is . . . their price! Thanks to marketing, hyaluronic acid has become a more coveted and therefore more expensive ingredient in skincare. Glycerin works just as well as hyaluronic acid and can be found in less expensive (yet still effective) skincare products. Some dermatologists favor glycerin since it naturally occurs in the skin's outermost layers, whereas hyaluronic acid is naturally found in deeper layers of the skin. So when we topically apply glycerin, we're actually replacing the molecule in the area where it's naturally found. But since hyaluronic acid is found deeper in the skin, applying it topically can never truly replenish it in the layer where it naturally occurs. The primary drawback of glycerin is that it can give a tacky residue to the skin. If you're particularly sensitive to that tackiness, you can reap the benefits of glycerin by incorporating it into your evening routine.

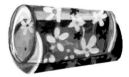

Squalane

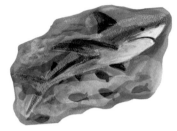

Also falls under **Plumping**

Your body's sebaceous glands create sebum, which makes up your body's natural sweat and oil. While you may have been taught to think that oil in skincare products is the enemy—just check the skincare aisle of your local drugstore for all the products that proudly proclaim themselves "oil-free"—in fact, your skin needs oil for optimum health. All the sebum that your body produces actually creates a protective layer of moisture on the outer layer of your skin. That sweat and oil is a cocktail of all kinds of natural fats, one of them being **squalene**. Now, squalene itself can't be extracted for topical uses—it's far too unstable to be stored in a bottle and used in skincare. But scientists realized that **squalane**, a derivative of squalene, actually can work in skincare products— and it's a damn good way of making sure your skin is thoroughly hydrated with a layer of intensely moisturizing fats. Squalane is not a humectant, so it doesn't draw moisture to itself. Instead, squalane is an emollient that seals in moisture and minimizes moisture loss, which is why it works great as a primary ingredient in products used in the final step in your routine, like moisturizers or face oils. It's safe for most skin types. Unfortunately, many brands source their squalane in unethical ways by extracting it from animals, namely sharks, who have more squalane in their bodies than any other animal on the planet. Thankfully, due to an increase in the public's concern for shark conservation, many companies have begun sourcing squalane through plant-based alternatives such as olives, rice bran, and wheat oil. In order to figure out if a squalane-containing product has been derived from animals, you can always reach out to the brand via social media or email and ask about their practices. Alternatively, seek out a vegan and cruelty-free brand.

Snail Mucin

Also falls under **Healing, Illuminating, Smoothing**, and **Plumping**

Okay, I know this sounds gross, but hear me out: mucin is the trail of excretion that snails leave behind as they move around. I wouldn't tell you to smear snail slime on your face if it weren't simply one of the best all-around ingredients on the market. Snail mucin is great for regenerating and hydrating the skin. It encourages collagen production, soothes the skin, helps repair damaged tissue, and,

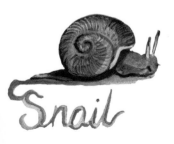

since it's composed of 91–98 percent water, effectively restores hydration. Snail mucin is used to treat a wide variety of conditions, including dry skin, wrinkles, acne, pigmentation, and bumps. Truth be told, the ethics behind how snail mucin is harvested are a bit ambiguous. Most brands claim that their mucin is collected in a nonharmful way, but some skeptics question whether the snails have actually been treated humanely throughout the harvesting process. If you're concerned or hoping to achieve an entirely plant based skincare routine, avoid snail mucin.

ILLUMINATING

Most people can benefit from using more illuminating products and ingredients in their routines. Whether you have acne and are hoping to eradicate the marks left behind from breakouts, or you're coming out of the winter months with extra-dull, "bleh"-looking skin, or you don't know what exactly your issues are—you just know you want to look glowier and less blotchy—the illuminating pillar is a great place to start. Unlike ingredients that fall under the hydrating category, which provide a kind of instant gratification (you can appear and feel more moisturized as soon as you apply a good moisturizer), ingredients that promise to add radiance, glowiness, or luminosity to your complexion often play the long game. This means you will need to implement them into your routine regularly, and it can often take weeks, if not months, to see results. But impatience aside, these ingredients can produce incredibly gratifying changes, which is why many have become skincare staples.

Niacinamide

Also falls under **Smoothing**, **Plumping**, **Healing**, and **Hydrating**
Can also be found in ingredient lists as
- *Vitamin B3*
- *Nicotinamide*

Niacinamide is a water-soluble vitamin—it won't dissolve in oil, so you'll typically find it in water-based serums. Niacinamide is known (and loved by many a skincare obsessive) for its ability to help manage acne, rosacea, hyperpigmentation, and textural issues. Studies show that niacinamide has sebum-controlling, wound-healing, and smoothing properties, making it a great choice for people suffering from acne. Niacinamide has the ability to restore and maintain the strength of the ceramides in the body, therefore helping the skin's surface fight against dehydration and moisture loss. There's some evidence of its ability to produce more collagen, elastin, and hyaluronic acid in the body, but it's better as an illuminating or smoothing treatment. Niacinamide is suitable for most skin types, except for particularly sensitive ones. Niacinamide is almost unique among other workhorse ingredients in its compatibility with most other popular skincare actives, including chemical exfoliators (AHAs and BHAs), retinoids, hyaluronic acid, and vitamin C (we'll get to all of these later).

I call ingredients like niacinamide "sidekicks"—they work well on their own, but used in conjunction with other ingredients, such as the ones just mentioned, they thrive. Niacinamide is an ingredient that I think most skincare lovers should try incorporating into their routine.

Vitamin C

Also falls under **Plumping** and **Healing**
Can also be found in ingredient lists as
    Water soluble:

- *Ascorbic acid*
- *Magnesium ascorbyl phosphate*

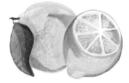

Lipid soluble:

- *Tetrahexyldecyl ascorbate*
- *Ascorbyl palmitate*
- *Glyceryl ascorbate*
- *Ester-C*

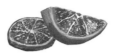

Plant extracts high in vitamin C:

- *Actinidia chinensis (Chinese kiwi)*
- *Hippophae rhamnoides (sea buckthorn)*

Vitamin C is a potent **antioxidant**: it is a chemical that comes in many different forms with a slew of different names and that helps prevent damage caused by free radicals and environmental stressors, such as pollution and UV rays. Like other antioxidants, it's not just preventative, but actually helps the skin repair damaged cells. Melanin, a natural pigment in the skin, determines the skin's natural color and—when affected by sun, inflammation, or hormonal changes—can create bruise-like or pinkish patches on the skin. Vitamin C contains a property that inhibits the skin's melanin overproduction and can help prevent PIE, PIH, and sun spots from forming, as well as fade old ones, while also protecting the skin from the harmful effects of sunburn-causing UVB rays.

There are lots of different forms of vitamin C in skincare, but the most widely studied and used form is the water-soluble ascorbic acid (chances are, if you've tried a few vitamin C serums, you've used one that contains this). But just because it's the most popular, it doesn't mean it's the only one available.

For people who like to have a more botanical-based skincare routine, plant extracts that contain a high percentage of vitamin C (like Chinese kiwi and sea buckthorn, for example) tend to be more appealing options. The primary issue with botanical formulas is that there tends to be some variability in the concentration—not every plant is created exactly equal, so some might contain more vitamin C than others.

Lipid-soluble forms of vitamin C, such as tetrahexyldecyl ascorbate, ascorbyl palmitate, glyceryl ascorbate, and Ester-C, are being incorporated into more formulas on the market. While they might not be as widely researched and used as ascorbic acid, lipid-soluble alternatives are actually favored by some researchers and skincare lovers. Some researchers believe lipid-soluble forms of vitamin C have a longer shelf life; ascorbic-acid formulas can expire *quickly* (more on that shortly), while lipid-soluble forms are more stable. Lipid-soluble formulas are also able to penetrate deeper into the skin than ascorbic acid—they can actually go into the dermis rather than just sitting on the surface of the skin. And, finally, since lipid-soluble formulas have a fatty acid base, they actually tend to be less sensitizing. If you have ever tried an ascorbic-acid-based vitamin C serum and had breakouts or irritation from it, you should consider trying a lipid-soluble vitamin C, such as tetrahexyldecyl ascorbate.

Expiration and Vitamin C

How long a vitamin C serum can last in your medicine cabinet is completely contingent on the bottle and formula. If it's an unstable formula and frequently exposed to light and air—if you don't screw the cap on well or if the bottle isn't opaque—it can go bad quickly. But if it's a more stable formula in airless packaging and stored airtight in a dark place, it can stay potent for years.

When a vitamin C product expires, it usually changes color, from clear or light orange to a darker brown. That's your signal that it's time to toss it and buy a new one.

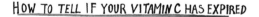

HOW TO TELL IF YOUR VITAMIN C HAS EXPIRED

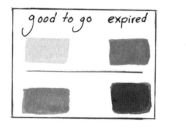

good to go   expired

Licorice Root Extract

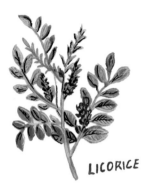

LICORICE

Also falls under **Healing**

Can also be found in ingredient lists as

- *Licorice root water*
- *Licorice root juice*
- *Licorice root powder*
- *Licorice leaf extract*

Licorice root extract is a gentle, natural illuminating ingredient, often recommended for extra-sensitive skin types. Some research has shown that licorice root extract can assist in combating and preventing sun damage and hyperpigmentation as it's rich in glabridin, an antioxidant that has both skin-soothing and radiance-boosting properties. There isn't as much research behind licorice root's ability to heal severe pigmentation issues, so vitamin C is still the dermatologist-preferred choice for those.

PLUMPING

As we age, our body's natural collagen and elastin (the elements that make skin firm, taut, and elastic) decrease, making it easier to develop fine lines and wrinkles around the eyes, forehead, and mouth.

I'd be remiss not to mention that there's something undoubtedly beautiful about the natural aging process—how these indentations are indicative of things we've done and seen, what we've accomplished in our lives. And while, as with any skin concern from wrinkles to acne, accepting your skin is one of the best things you can do to feel better mentally, the desire to treat your skin with kindness by helping it build strength and vitality doesn't necessarily mean you don't love it.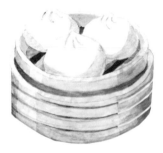

Plumping, as it will be discussed in this section, goes hand in hand with hydrating. Most plumping ingredients can't truly do their work on a molecular level without the added assistance of moisture, which works as an additional cushion or sealant. This is why you'll notice that most products that promise to plump your skin also lock in moisture.

Ceramides

Also falls under **Hydrating**, **Healing**, and **Smoothing**
Can be found in ingredient lists as
- *Phytosphingosine*
- *Sphingolipids*

Ceramides are the naturally occurring fatty lipids in our body that help us maintain buoyancy and vitality in our skin. They're also a part of the skin's barrier, so they help protect the skin against free radicals caused by environmental stressors such as weather or pollution. Ceramides help keep the skin hydrated and nourished and are also capable of preventing textural issues as well as reducing irritation and redness. Much like hyaluronic acid, ceramides decrease in our body as we age. So replenishing the skin with ceramide-rich formulas can help restore that bounce and plumpness. Vitamin F, an ingredient revered for its skin-plumping, moisture-locking, and protective capabilities, helps create ceramides in the skin when applied topically.

Peptides

Also falls under **Hydrating** and **Healing**

Can also be found in ingredient lists as

- *Marine algae*

Peptides are short chains of amino acids that naturally plump up and moisturize your skin. When peptides are applied to the skin, they act as little messengers that trigger the skin cells to start building collagen and elastin, making the skin appear firmer and therefore bouncier. Peptides are wonderful, but they should be applied alongside antioxidants such as vitamin C or retinol, as they cannot alone protect skin from free radicals, the particles that cause premature aging (such as collagen breakdown and wrinkles). Peptides can also signal the body to make more hyaluronic acid, which is why they can also be found under the hydrating pillar.

What's a Free Radical?

Free radicals are unstable molecules that our bodies generate from pollution, UV rays, cigarettes, alcohol, pesticides, or preservatives in processed foods. These molecules attack our cells and trigger premature aging. Antioxidants stabilize, and therefore combat, these molecules.

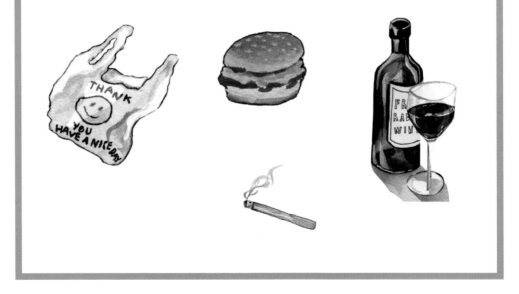

HEALING

People who suffer from consistent eczema, rosacea, or blemish-related redness or inflammation, as well as anyone who has trouble with skin picking or frequent wounds, can benefit from the ingredients listed in this category. Users of acid exfoliators or retinoids, too, can benefit from using healing ingredients to achieve added anti-inflammatory benefits while also preventing these intense treatments from stripping or drying out their skin.

Propolis

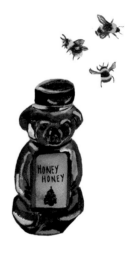

Also falls under **Plumping**, **Smoothing**, and **Hydrating**
Propolis is a concoction of beeswax and pollen used by honeybees to protect and coat the walls of their hives. Propolis is believed to have healing, antiseptic, and restorative capabilities, which can soothe any kind of blemish, scab, or irritation. Some believe it can also accelerate the rate of cell turnover, unclog pores, protect the skin against bacterial growth, and function as a moisturizing agent.

Green Tea

Also falls under **Hydrating, Illuminating,** and **Plumping**

Can also be found in ingredient lists as

- *Camellia sinensis*

Green tea is rich in antioxidants and amino acids that can help relieve skin irritation, inflammation, and redness while helping smooth textural issues and hydrate the skin. Studies have shown that green tea can help soothe, calm, and even fade away damage from UV rays, as well as inflamed breakouts and irritation. Green tea is safe for most skin types, but is particularly suitable for those with sensitive skin, rosacea, or acne-prone skin.

Centella Asiatica

Also falls under **Hydrating** and **Smoothing**

Can also be found in ingredient lists as

- *Centella asiatica leaf water*
- *Cica*
- *Asiatic pennywort*
- *Tiger grass*
- *Gotu kola*

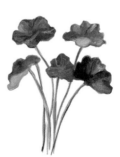

Centella asiatica is said to boost antioxidant activity at the site of wounds, strengthening the skin and increasing blood circulation. It is beneficial in the management of eczema, psoriasis, and varicose veins (visibly enlarged or swollen veins). Certain *Centella* extracts have been shown to have antibacterial and antifungal properties. For acne sufferers, it speeds healing, helping to prevent scarring and future blemishes. It also has been shown to have hydrating and nourishing properties.

Panthenol

Also falls under **Illuminating** and **Hydrating**
Can also be found in ingredient lists as
- *Dexpanthenol*
- *D-pantothenyl*
- *Butanamide*
- *Provitamin B5*

Panthenol has been shown to improve hydration and reduce itching and inflammation of the skin, so it's suitable for eczema- and rosacea-prone skin types. Some research shows that it can speed up and improve the healing of wounds on the epidermis (the top layer of skin), which is why it's often used in sunburn-treatment products. Panthenol is also a humectant, an ingredient that attracts and holds water in the skin, making it excellent for hydration as well.

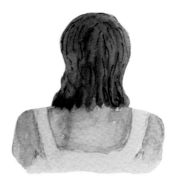

Mugwort

Also falls under **Smoothing** and **Hydrating**

Mugwort is a weed commonly used in both Korean cuisine and medicine that has antibacterial, antifungal, moisturizing, and skin-healing properties. This antioxidant-rich weed is known to have calming and soothing effects on any kind of inflamed, angry, or hot skin. Mugwort is a great ingredient to look

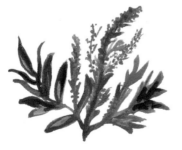

out for if you are looking to reduce the redness or swelling of any active or healing blemishes or to diminish redness from environmental stressors, irritation, or rosacea. You're most likely to find this ingredient in soothing sheet masks and essences.

Tea Tree Oil

Also falls under **Smoothing**

Can also be found in ingredient lists as

- *Melaleuca oil*

Tea tree oil is one of the most commonly known and trusted methods of treating inflammation. It has antibacterial, antifungal, anti-inflammatory, and antioxidant properties that help reduce the size and redness of breakouts or irritation. While pure tea tree oil can leave your skin at risk for sensitization or dryness, it is diluted in most tea tree products for calming and anti-inflammatory benefits with less risk of drying out your skin.

Vitamin E

Also falls under **Hydrating** and **Plumping**

Can also be found in ingredient lists as

- *Tocopheryl acetate*
- *Tocopherol*

Vitamin E is a powerful, fat-soluble antioxidant that naturally occurs within our bodies, but can also be found in fatty foods such as nuts and seeds. Its healing and skin-repairing properties can help with anything from burns to scars to sun damage and can also help reduce redness and swelling from breakouts or irritation. Due to its antioxidant properties, it helps strengthen the barrier that protects skin from environmental stressors like air pollution and sun damage. Though most evidence is still anecdotal, Vitamin E is a go-to ingredient that many rely on to heal and repair things like burns, scars, or sun damage.

SMOOTHING

Smoothing ingredients are best suited for those who struggle with acne and/or textural issues—whether that be mild, once-a-month pimples, more frequently occurring cystic clusters, or simply bumpy, rough skin. While many smoothing ingredients are meant to target and control the main causes of acne and refine uneven skin texture, high concentrations of certain ingredients, like salicylic acid or benzoyl peroxide, can be particularly harsh on the skin, creating irritation that triggers further breakouts and roughness. When it comes to these ingredients, it's good to reach for lower concentrations (about

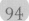

5 percent and under for AHAs, 1 percent and under for BHAs) for more frequent use (two or three times a week) or higher concentrations (about 10–15 percent AHA) for less frequent treatments (once every week or two). When used properly, with restraint, these ingredients can be some of the most effective acne-fighting tools in your arsenal.

Exfoliators

In part three, I'm going to deep dive into the world of exfoliators: what they are, what they do, and how they work. But just for a little bit of context, exfoliators are skincare ingredients that can help buff away dead skin cells, revealing smoother and more radiant skin, and treat a bevy of skin issues, from sun spots to post-inflammatory hyperpigmentation to acne.

Acids? On Your Face?

When it comes to exfoliating, there are three major classes of acid exfoliators on the market: alpha hydroxy acids (AHAs), beta hydroxy acids (BHAs), and polyhydroxy acids (PHAs), each with different uses. AHAs (such as lactic, glycolic, malic, citric, mandelic, and tartaric acids) exfoliate the skin's surface, so they're great for helping reduce flakiness caused by dehydrated or sun-damaged skin and resurfacing textural issues. BHAs (such as salicylic acid) have anti-inflammatory and antibacterial properties, penetrating deeper down to combat breakouts, enlarged pores, and blackheads. PHAs (such as gluconolactone, galactose, and lactobionic acids) are much larger and therefore much gentler than AHAs and BHAs. They are humectants, meaning they attract water, and do most of their work on the very surface of the skin. Their molecular size and moisturizing capabilities make them less harsh than AHAs and BHAs, so they are an excellent choice for people with very sensitive skin types who still want mild exfoliation. Some skincare enthusiasts are loyal to one or another, but many products use a low concentration of AHAs, BHAs, and PHAs in order to ensure you're getting all the benefits of chemical exfoliators. Since exfoliators help remove dead skin cells, they can also increase sun sensitivity, which is why daily sunscreen application is *extra* important when you're using exfoliating products.

AHAs	BHAs	PHAs
Glycolic acid	Salicylic acid	Gluconolactone acid
Lactic acid		Galactose acid
Mandelic acid		Lactobionic acid
Tartaric acid		
Malic acid		
Citric acid		

Lactic Acid

Also falls under **Illuminating**, **Plumping**, and **Hydrating**

Can also be found in ingredient lists as

- *Ammonium lactate*

Lactic acid is an AHA that helps exfoliate the skin's surface by breaking down and removing the "glue" that holds dead skin cells together. It's a great ingredient for treating textural issues, as it works to unclog built-up skin cells around hair follicles. Lactic acid treatments can help smooth bumps from acne, closed comedones, eczema, and even keratosis pilaris (commonly known as "chicken skin" and often found on arms). Lactic acid is also known to help with surface-level skin issues such as hyperpigmentation and sun spots, as well as mild fine lines and wrinkles (for a deeper treatment, you may want to try retinoids). Lactic acid is a larger molecule than glycolic acid (meaning it naturally can't penetrate as deeply), so it is often seen as a better option for those with sensitive skin. Unlike other AHAs, lactic acid can also stimulate ceramides in the skin, giving it moisturizing properties that are ideal for drier skin types. Lactic acid occurs naturally in foods like milk and yogurt, but it is also created synthetically in labs for stability purposes.

Glycolic Acid

Also falls under **Illuminating** and **Plumping**
Can also be found in ingredient lists as
  - *Ammonium glycolate*
  - *Sodium glycolate*

Glycolic acid is one of the most widely used AHAs in skincare. It helps remove the sealant that keeps skin cells together and encourages dead skin cells to fall off faster. While glycolic acid works in a similar way as its AHA siblings (mandelic and lactic acids), it has a smaller molecular size that allows for deeper penetration—it can reach the hair follicles and loosen up collected debris (such as sebum and proteins) that might lead to breakouts. It adds radiance to the complexion by pulling off the dead skin cells that store excess pigment from sun damage and/or hyperpigmentation, and it is even known to have collagen-stimulating benefits. When used correctly, glycolic acid can be suitable for a wide range of skin types. However, it can be irritating, particularly on dry or sensitive skin types, when used excessively.

Mandelic Acid

Also falls under **Illuminating** and **Plumping**
Can also be found in ingredient lists as
- *Amygdalic acid*

Mandelic acid has the largest molecular size of all the AHAs, which means it's the most gentle option for sensitive skin types. It has both exfoliating and antibacterial capabilities, making it a great choice for those who suffer from textural issues and/or acne. As a milder exfoliant, mandelic acid is often used in conjunction with other treatments, rather than as a stand-alone ingredient. For example, a common chemical-peel treatment for patients with mild to moderate acne is 45 percent mandelic acid and 30 percent salicylic acid. Mandelic acid is also known to help even out complexions (a study showed it can help reduce hyperpigmentation in melasma) and stimulate collagen, softening the appearance of fine lines and wrinkles.

Salicylic Acid

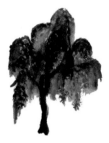

Can also be found in ingredient lists as
- *Willow bark extract*

Salicylic acid, a BHA exfoliator, is derived from willow bark. It is an exfoliating treatment that helps break down and dissolve the skin debris that clogs pores. Salicylic acid has extreme smoothing and anti-inflammatory properties, which makes it a great choice for acne-prone skin. But as it is a strong exfoliator, it should be used either in very low dosages or higher dosages less frequently. Particularly for dry or sensitive skin types, overuse of salicylic acid can create an overproduction of oil to compensate for dehydration, inadvertently causing irritation and more breakouts. While salicylic acid is better for oily skin types, those with dry skin who suffer from acne can incorporate it in their routine so long as they look for a product that contains a low percentage of salicylic acid (less than 1 percent for leave-on treatments, and 2 percent for wash-off treatments, like cleansers), as well as more hydrating ingredients, such as glycerin, that can help make the treatment less aggressive on the skin.

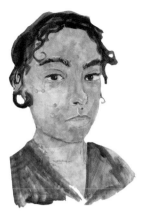

Benzoyl Peroxide

Benzoyl peroxide is a chemical that dives deep into pores to kill bacteria within the skin, helping to reduce the size and redness of acne. Though it works on all kinds of acne, it's more noticeably effective as a spot treatment on pustules and papules. A higher percentage of benzoyl peroxide can irritate the skin, especially if you are on the sensitive side. A lower percentage, such as 2 percent or less, is more than enough to effectively treat the skin without causing serious irritation.

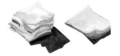

Retinoids

Also falls under **Illuminating** and **Plumping**

Can also be found in ingredient lists as

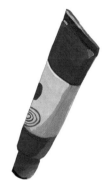

- *Retinol*
- *Adapalene (generic for Differin)*
- *Retin-A*
- *Tretinoin (generic for Retin-A)*
- *Tazarotene (generic for Tazorac)*

Retinoids are some of the most intensely effective and widely studied skincare ingredients on the market. The word *retinoid* actually serves as an umbrella term for a few different products, all of which use vitamin A to promote an increase in cell turnover. Retinoids not only encourage skin to build collagen and elastin, but they also exfoliate and treat acne by increasing cell turnover to unclog and open up pores. While they start working immediately, you won't see results for about six weeks, so be patient. Prescription retinoid formulas are significantly stronger than over the counter, so you'll see more intense results quicker—smoother, more radiant, and more even skin—with a potentially heightened purging and shedding period.

Purging Might Happen! And That's Okay!

While the stellar results of retinoids have been proven time and again, retinoids (particularly prescription-strength ones) do have a tendency to sensitize the skin, causing increased breakouts, dryness, tightness, and irritation, a process called **purging**. Since retinoids essentially encourage your skin to push new skin cells to the surface, your skin can become flaky and tender as it adjusts to this new, sped-up cycle of regeneration. In the process, it's also pushing all the gunk that might currently be in your pores to the surface, which is why it's common to see breakouts when you first start using retinoids. Purging can last anywhere from a week to a few weeks when you first integrate a retinoid into your routine—while that might seem like forever in the moment, it is worth it for the incredible results you'll see afterwards.

Another common reaction for first-time users is "retinoid dermatitis"—redness, flaking, or skin sensitivity that's often seen in response to more concentrated or medical-grade retinoids. While all skin types are susceptible to retinoid dermatitis, those with particularly sensitive skin types are extra prone to it.

Retinol can be found in many over-the-counter products, like night creams, eye creams, and serums. Retin-A, on the other hand, is found exclusively in prescription medication and has the ability to aid in the treatment of acne as well as fine lines and wrinkles.

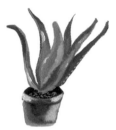

WHAT TO DO, WHAT NOT TO DO

Throughout this part, we've discussed common skincare ingredients—how they interact with your skin and when you should reach for them. Now, let's shift our attention to what you should avoid: the ingredients that will make your products aggravating or less effective.

Ingredients People with Acne-Prone or Sensitive Skin Should Consider Avoiding

These ingredients can deteriorate your skin's acid mantle, which is the natural protective barrier within your skin:

Alcohol, listed also as *denatured alcohol, ethyl alcohol,* or *isopropyl alcohol*

Fragrance, listed also as *parfum*

Sulfates, listed as *sodium lauryl sulfate* or *sodium laureth sulfate*

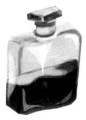

"Fragrance"

The FDA doesn't require brands to disclose what constitutes the fragrances in their products because they are technically considered to be a brand's trade secrets. The downside for consumers is that this secrecy gives brands the opportunity to hide ingredients (like potential allergens or irritants) under the umbrella of "fragrance." To avoid this loophole, steer clear of anything that has *perfume*, *parfum*, or *fragrance* listed in the ingredients. Importantly, just because a product has *unscented* on the label does not mean it's actually fragrance-free. In fact, this generally means that the formula includes an artificial masking ingredient that covers up the smell of the product's ingredients (this is often used when a product contains ingredients that smell bad, "chemically," or just generally very potent). "Fragrance-free," on the other hand, means the product was formulated with no masking scents or fragrance material.

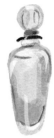

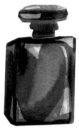

Though it's often vilified in skincare, the truth is not *everyone* is sensitive to fragrance. In fact, I know tons of skincare experts who

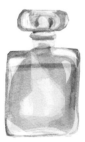

don't mind it in small concentrations in their formulas. But if you're very sensitive, break out easily, and/or have had a bad reaction to a fragranced product in the past, I understand wanting to avoid all fragrance to the best of your ability.

What's the Deal with Essential Oils?

Synthetic fragrances are made with chemicals in a lab while natural fragrances are derived from plant-based aromatics. Essential oils—such as lavender oil, rosemary oil, and clary sage oil—are considered natural fragrances. Like synthetic fragrances, they are capable of triggering skin irritation. But at very low concentrations, they can also benefit the skin by delivering antibacterial or antioxidant properties. While someone with particularly sensitive or acne-prone skin might want to avoid essential oils altogether, formulas that use them at minimal concentrations don't need to be avoided at all costs. If you own a product that contains small amounts of natural fragrance and you haven't had any bad reactions from it, it's okay to continue using it.

Alcohol

Not *all* alcohol is bad for your complexion. Some (like cetyl and cetearyl alcohol) are fatty alcohols, which can actually help products become creamier and more hydrating on the skin. However, if you see denatured alcohol, isopropyl alcohol, or ethyl alcohol listed, stay away—these can be extremely drying, stripping, and irritating.

DON'TS

People have a tendency to think that more skincare products means better results. In fact, piling lots of products on top of one another can lead to further skin irritation. We'll talk in the next part about how to properly layer products to ensure their maximum effectiveness, but here's a cheat sheet of a few ingredients that shouldn't ever be used together.

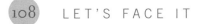

Retinoids and Vitamin C

There's long been a myth that, when used together, vitamin C and retinoids cancel each other out due to their drastically different pH levels (vitamin C generally works at less than pH 3.5 and retinoids around pH 5.5–6). In fact, this is not true. Retinoids and vitamin C remain totally stable and effective when used together and can even increase each other's illuminating, smoothing, and collagen-building capabilities. However, since both ingredients can be sensitizing, I personally recommend using them during different parts of your routine. I like to use vitamin C in the morning and retinoids in the evening to avoid irritating my temperamental skin.

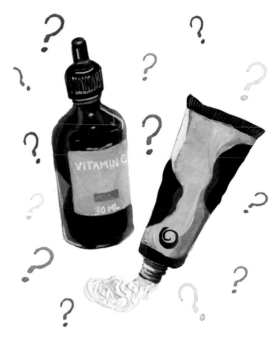

pH Levels

The pH level is a measurement of how acidic or alkaline a certain substance is—14 being the most alkaline (or basic) and 0 being the most acidic. The natural pH of skin is about 5.5, fairly neutral leaning slightly acidic.

Being aware of your skin's pH level is a great way to maintain optimal skin health. A drop or increase in your pH level (often the result of harsh or stripping skincare products) can disrupt your acid mantle, making your skin more susceptible to damage. Breakouts, irritation, and redness are common side effects of pH imbalance. You can correct a pH imbalance by skipping harsh treatments for a while and sticking to gentle hydrating or healing ingredients until your skin returns to normal.

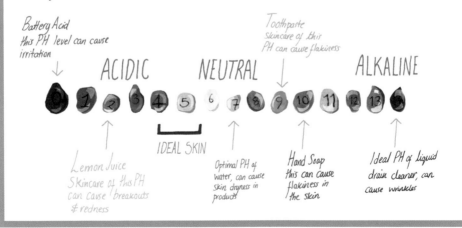

Battery Acid
this PH level can cause irritation

ACIDIC

Toothpaste
skincare of this PH can cause flakiness

NEUTRAL

ALKALINE

IDEAL SKIN

Lemon Juice
Skincare of this PH can cause breakouts & redness

Optimal PH of water, can cause skin dryness in products

Hand Soap
this can cause flakiness in the skin

Ideal PH of liquid drain cleaner, can cause wrinkles

What's an Acid Mantle?

The acid mantle is a thin, acidic film on the surface of the skin that helps protect the skin from viruses, bacteria, and environmental stressors.

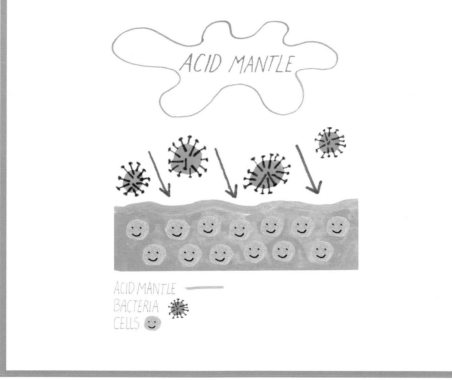

Retinoids with AHAs and BHAs

Just thinking about this makes my skin irritated! AHAs, BHAs, and retinoids are three of the most intensive at-home treatments you can use on your skin. Overuse of any of these products on their own can create a lot of irritation, but using them all at the same time can trigger an enormous eruption of sensitivity and redness. In order to have all of these products in your arsenal at once, you need to split them up: I recommend alternating between using exfoliators (AHAs and BHAs) for a month and retinoids for a month. Or you can rotate them every week.

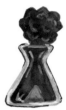

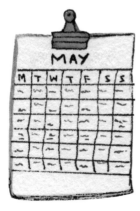

AHAs, PHAs, and BHAs

Some products have a blend of both AHAs and BHAs or AHAs and PHAs at low concentrations, specifically formulated so that your skin is able to safely achieve multiple kinds of exfoliation. You should not, however, apply different exfoliating products from your medicine cabinet in the same day, let alone in the same routine. You should use only one exfoliating product in your routine per day; otherwise you can strip your skin and cause dehydration and irritation.

DO'S

Sunscreen and Vitamin C

One of the most magical combinations in skincare is sunscreen and vitamin C. Vitamin C is proven to increase sunscreen's ability to protect the skin from UVB rays. While vitamin C won't shield the skin from harmful UVB rays when applied alone, the extra boost of protection from vitamin C strengthens your sunscreen's ability to do its job.

Glycerin and Retinoids

It's common to experience irritation, redness, and dryness when you first incorporate retinoids into your routine. Glycerin can help ease that dryness and irritation by delivering water to your parched skin. This takes the edge off of the severity of the retinoid's transitional period without disturbing its activity.

SUNSCREEN

You may be wondering why we haven't yet talked about sunscreen. While sunscreen has some of the most powerful firming, illuminating, and protective benefits of any type of product on the market, I also believe that it has its own set of rules to take 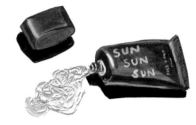 into account when selecting one that's right for you. Put simply, a good sunscreen should be the very heart of any skincare routine. Without it, your skin will constantly be susceptible to damage from the sun, and all the vitamin C serums and ceramide-rich creams in the world won't help. You can't repair something that's constantly being damaged, right?

We've been taught to apply sunscreen when we're spending long hours at the beach or lying in the park on a sunny day, but we get more inadvertent sun exposure on a daily basis than you think. For example, when you're sitting at your desk or driving in your car, UVA rays are capable of penetrating through your windows. Even a quick run to the grocery store can be surprisingly damaging.

Finding the sunscreen formula that's best for you can sometimes require a bit of trial and error. We'll talk more about sunscreens in part three, but here's a bit of information on the two types of sunscreens and how their ingredients and formulas differ.

Chemical vs. Physical Sunscreens

There are two different kinds of sunscreens: chemical and physical. The active ingredients in chemical sunscreens work by absorbing the sun's UV rays, converting them to heat before they can damage your skin's DNA (which causes premature aging and increases your risk of skin cancer). People who are looking to avoid white casts (the pallor that thick sunscreens can sometimes give you) prefer chemical sunscreens, as they tend to have more lightweight formulas and are better for sitting underneath makeup.

Physical sunscreens, also known as mineral sunscreens, protect the skin by creating a barrier that helps block UV rays. However, some new research shows that physical sunscreens also absorb UV rays and convert them to heat.

Both chemical and physical sunscreen should be applied about fifteen to twenty minutes before going outside.

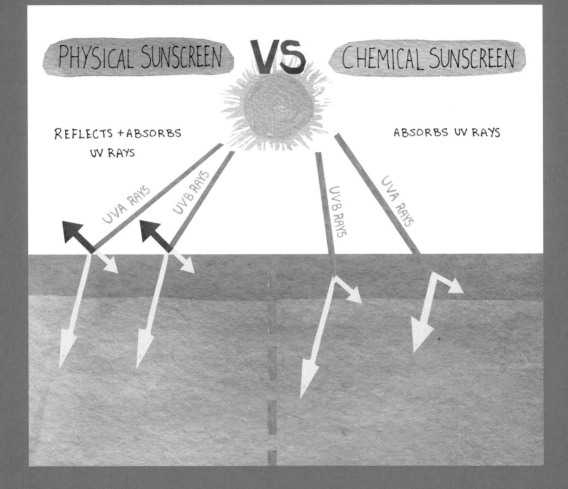

How to Tell Whether a Sunscreen Is Chemical or Physical

Sunscreens are considered an over-the-counter drug by the FDA, so all sunscreens are required to include a box on the packaging of "Drug Facts," which lists their active ingredients.

Active Ingredients in Physical Sunscreens

Zinc oxide

Titanium dioxide

Common Active Ingredients in Chemical Sunscreens

Oxybenzone

Avobenzone

Octisalate

Octocrylene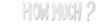

Homosalate

Octinoxate

We've spent a lot of time thinking about the science behind ingredients. But now, it's time to explore how to actually use them in skincare. In the next part, we'll dive into the vast and overwhelming landscape of products—everything from toners to essences to eye creams—and learn what they actually do and how to pick the best ones for you.

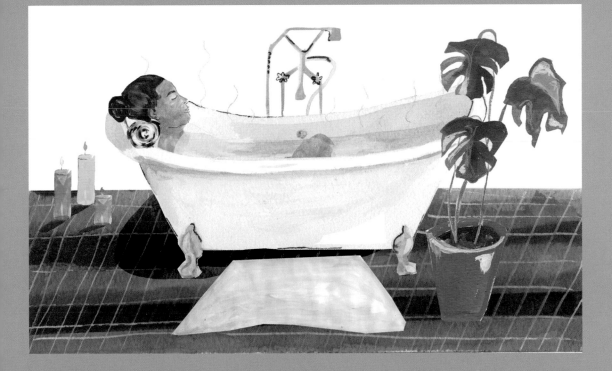

PART THREE

Serums, Potions, and More

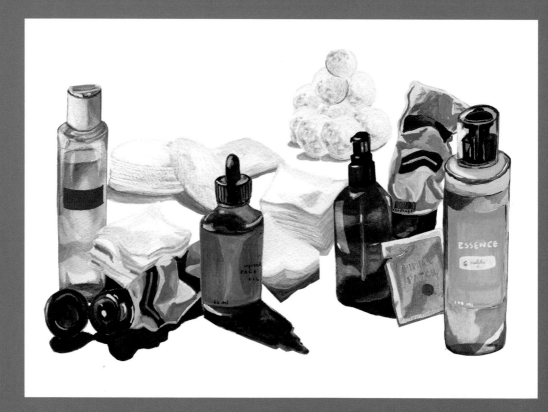

My hope is that in the previous parts, you've familiarized yourself with the pillars of skincare—you have a greater understanding of how ingredients interact with your skin and a stronger sense of what to avoid and look out for. Now, let's discuss the products that all those ingredients come packaged in. You may have heard, either with admiration or an eye roll, about celebrities, influencers, or estheticians with skincare routines so elaborate their products number in the double digits. But, before you shut this book in alarm, I want to assure you that it's entirely possible to create an effective routine without having to layer a ton of products every single day. Yes, some people may see positive results from an extensive, lengthy routine, but other people may experience the exact same level of satisfaction from only two or three steps. In this part, we'll be building a routine specifically for you and your lifestyle—not the beauty editor you follow on Instagram whose medicine cabinet is jam packed, not your know-it-all, skincare-obsessed friend . . . you! We want to create a routine that you'll realistically incorporate into your daily life.

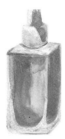

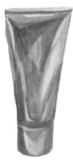

Just like Charlotte Cho's vision for the ten-step K-beauty (that's "Korean beauty" for short) routine, the steps described in this part are here to serve as a model for layering. They're a guidebook to help you apply multiple products in a particular order to ensure maximum effectiveness. This is not a universal skincare model to which everyone must strictly adhere in order to achieve clear skin. Ultimately, it's an educational tool used to explain what specific products are doing for your skin and how they should be applied for the best results.

If you're just starting to create a routine, or if you're uncertain about how the products you currently use are working for you, start by paring those back to three products at most: a cleanser, a serum or moisturizer, and sunscreen, used in that order. Then, after a week, once you understand how your skin is responding to those three products, you can—if you want—begin to incorporate more steps, adding products one by one. That way, you'll be able to tell the exact effects of each product—and if one causes a bad reaction, you'll know exactly who the culprit is, avoiding a time-consuming and stressful whodunit. Even as someone who works in beauty, and whose job it is to test and try as many products as possible, I limit myself to testing two new products a month, to avoid any surprises.

Understanding the purpose of each step is vital to curating products that are right for your skin. While no product is created equal, some steps are geared towards specific pillars of skincare. For example, essences, moisturizers, sheet masks, face oils, and hydrating toners replenish, nourish, and moisturize the skin, which is why you'll notice lots of hydrating, healing, and plumping ingredients in their formulas. Vitamin C serums, exfoliators, and retinoids seek to resurface, refine, and restore your complexion, which is why you'll find ingredients that fall under the illuminating and smoothing pillar. Other products, like cleansers, serums, and wash-off masks have such a wide range of purposes, you should examine their ingredients to understand what they do. In this part, you will discover everything you need to choose the steps that are best suited for you and your skin type.

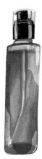

Most people apply their skincare products twice a day: once in the morning, to get ready for the day, and once at night, to cleanse the skin and help restore it overnight. Typically, your morning routine should be curated to protect you from the outside world: antioxidants, such as vitamin C, and sunscreen will help ensure that your skin is at its most resilient before going up against harsh environmental stressors like UV rays, wind, and pollution. Your evening routine should be composed mostly of

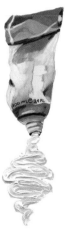

THE SKINCARE STEPS

HOW TO LAYER EVERYTHING PROPERLY

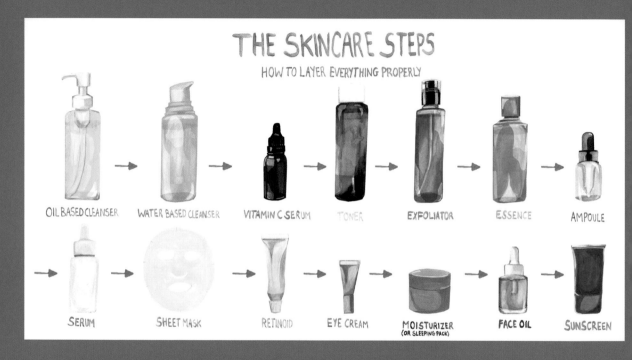

OIL BASED CLEANSER → WATER BASED CLEANSER → VITAMIN C SERUM → TONER → EXFOLIATOR → ESSENCE → AMPOULE

→ SERUM → SHEET MASK → RETINOID → EYE CREAM → MOISTURIZER (OR SLEEPING PACK) → FACE OIL → SUNSCREEN

deep, restorative treatments. Your skin does most of its repairing at night while you sleep, so making sure you're targeting your core skin issues before bed is important. Your evening routine is also when I encourage you to apply any chemical exfoliators or retinoids; that way, you can ensure they're not leaving your skin extra susceptible to sun damage while you're out and about during the day.

CLEANSERS

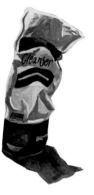

Cleansing is the first step in any skincare routine. Making sure your face is clear of makeup, sunscreen, dirt, sweat, or any other debris (including teeny-tiny pollutants that can penetrate into the skin) is essential for avoiding breakouts and irritated skin. Double cleansing is a two-step face-washing process that ensures your skin is as clean as possible. However, since the core intention of the two-part cleanse is to remove any makeup or sunscreen, even the most extreme skincare lovers usually opt out of double cleansing in the morning. For morning routines, some people, like me, use a neutral, cream-based cleanser to gently wash away any sweat from tossing and turning all night (I'm a sweaty sleeper! Gross, but honest). But other sensitive-skinned skincare experts swear by just splashing their face with some lukewarm or cold water in the morning, rinsing off any surface-level grime without stripping the skin.

At night, the traditional double cleanse begins with lathering an oil-based cleanser onto dry skin. Without any water, the oil is able to easily break down and dissolve any dirt or makeup that's collected on the surface of your skin throughout the day. As you rinse with cold or lukewarm water, enjoy watching the muddy concoction of mascara, grit, and concealer melt away.

Then, on wet skin, follow up with a water-based cleanser—this will eliminate any leftover dirt, sweat, or grime.

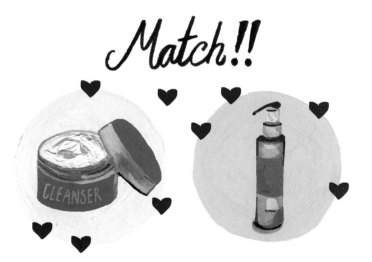

Why Cold Water?

Hot water can actually be quite dehydrating, as it pulls out the moisture from your pores. Cold or lukewarm water, on the other hand, is not only less drying, but it can also be a great way to wake yourself up in the morning.

Something that's always amused me is how often people believe they're exempt from the benefits of double cleansing. Here are just a few excuses I've heard over the years: "My skin is too dry to double cleanse," "I don't wear makeup so I don't need to double cleanse," "I'm acne prone, so I shouldn't use an oil cleanser." But the truth is, most skin types have something to gain from the double cleanse. No matter your skin type, there's a duo that can properly clean your skin without stripping it of its lovely natural oils. And it's not just for us daily makeup wearers—double cleansing is the most effective way to sanitize your skin from the grime, pollution, and sweat of the day. If you don't double cleanse, it's possible that you're letting all of that bacteria sink into your pores, which can lead to breakouts and irritation. And if you're opting out of a double cleanse because your makeup wipe is easier to use: I hate to break it to you, but makeup wipes are far less effective at removing makeup than a double cleanse and can be extremely irritating and stripping on the skin!

An easy way to check if your cleansers are right for you is to see how your skin feels immediately after washing it with your second cleanser and patting it dry. If it's tight, overly matte, and even a little painful to move your mouth, your cleansers are *way* too stripping for you. If it feels bouncy and soft to the touch, it's just right. People with irritated, dry, or dehydrated skin tend to prefer a creamy or milky formula for their second step, as it delivers more hydrating benefits. If your skin still feels shiny or oily after cleansing, you might want to gravitate towards foams and gels, which give the skin a deeper cleanse, for the second step.

DUAL CLEANSING CHEAT SHEET		
Oily skin types:	(1) micellar water or oil or balm cleanser	(2) gel cleanser or foam cleanser
Dry or sensitive skin types:	(1) micellar water or oil or balm cleanser	(2) cream or milk cleanser
Normal or combination skin types:	(1) micellar water or oil or balm cleanser	(2) gel cleanser

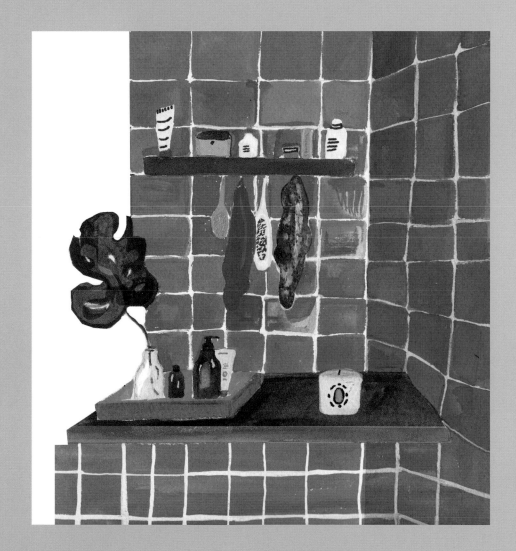

Step-One Cleansers

These cleansers are formulated to be the first product you apply to your skin and to help break down and dissolve surface-level dirt, debris, or makeup.

MICELLAR WATERS

In the past few years, micellar waters have become a popular alternative to the traditional oil-based first cleanse. Micellar water is a cleansing water product that uses a low-level surfactant (emulsifying agent) to remove surface-level dirt and debris left over from the day. The major benefit of micellar water is its convenience—you apply it to dry skin with a cotton round and don't need to rinse it off before continuing with your second cleanse. When purchasing a micellar water, make sure that alcohol and fragrances are not high up on the ingredient list; otherwise, it actually might be quite stripping and irritating. While many swear by micellar waters, I personally prefer oil cleansers, as I think they're more effective at removing heavy sweat and makeup.

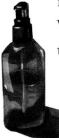

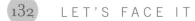

OIL AND BALM CLEANSERS

Both oil and balm cleansers are oil-based products, best at removing surface-level dirt and grime from the skin. The biggest distinction between oil and balm cleansers is in the texture of the product. A cleansing oil looks like a cooking oil—runny and liquidy—and is typically kept in a pump bottle. Balm cleansers, on the other hand, are usually kept in a jar, take a more solid form, and often come with a spatula for application. Generally, balm cleansers are less messy and more convenient for travel. Cleansing oils, however, are easier to use—a pump application is less of an ordeal than a spatula. Both oil and balm cleansers are suitable for all skin types, including oily and acne prone.

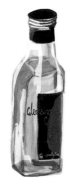

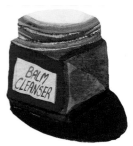

Step-Two Cleansers

The cleansers in step two are formulated to give your skin a more thorough cleanse. While they might not be as effective at removing your foundation or mascara from the day, they're wonderful as a second step to ensure your skin is as clean as possible before bed.

FOAM CLEANSERS

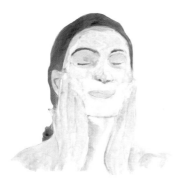

Foam cleansers are best for deep cleaning, making them excellent candidates for anyone with oily, acne-prone skin. However, foam cleansers sometimes include the ingredients sodium lauryl sulfate (SLS) or sodium laureth sulfate (SLES), which are sulfate-based surfactants that produce the product's sudsy, foamy texture. These ingredients can be stripping and are known to dry out and irritate sensitive, dry, rosacea-prone, or eczema-prone skin. But more foam cleansers are now being formulated with other milder or amino-rich surfactants such as sodium lauroyl sarcosinate, which can help achieve that sudsy effect in a less aggressive, stripping way. As we established in the previous section, not all products are created equal, so be sure to check the ingredient list before making a purchase.

CREAM AND MILK CLEANSERS

Cream and milk cleansers are typically made with an emulsion of fats and water, which is why they're often recommended for dry or ultra-sensitive skin types. A good cream or milk cleanser will clean your skin while ensuring it remains hydrated and pH balanced. The main distinction between cream and milk cleansers is in their consistency: milks tend to be a little more runny and liquidy.

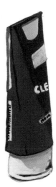

GEL CLEANSERS

Gel cleansers are great options for normal, combination, and oily skin types. They have a bouncy, gelatinous texture and typically provide a deeper, more purifying cleanse to the skin than milk or cream cleansers.

POWDER CLEANSERS

These cleansers take a powder form and are activated and transformed into a soft cream when water is added. These cleansers are suitable for all skin types and are especially convenient for travel.

TONERS

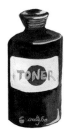

Toners have evolved with the expansion and increased sophistication of the skincare industry. The drugstore toners of my teen years were astringent, stripping, and claimed to combat acne by absorbing excess oil with harsh ingredients. But today, toners have developed into much more advanced and elegant products, with formulas versatile enough to target all skin concerns. Put simply, toners are liquid treatments that further cleanse, balance, and treat the skin and prep it for the rest of your routine.

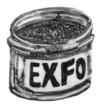

Hydrating Toners

The two most popular types of toners on the market are hydrating and exfoliating toners (more on exfoliators-slash-toners in a second). Hydrating toners are nourishing, pH-balancing liquid formulas that help replenish any moisture lost from your cleansing step and can also ensure any impurities left over from your cleanse are wiped off the skin.

EXFOLIATORS

Your skin is constantly turning over skin cells and leaving dead, old ones behind to collect on top of your skin. Exfoliating products help us do "housekeeping" against that buildup, in turn revealing a smooth and radiant surface beneath. If you suffer from acne, exfoliating can be one of the most helpful defense mechanisms against new breakouts. A buildup of dead skin cells on the surface of your skin can lead to clogged pores, which can trigger painful and irritating acne flare-ups. Exfoliating products not only buff away dead skin, but they can also expel bacteria from under the skin so that sebum can't gradually build up and create zits. If you suffer from acne, you likely suffer from hyperpigmentation as well—the discoloration or scarring that zits leave behind once they are no longer active. By removing that dead skin, exfoliating products also promote cell turnover, speeding up the healing of those PIE, PIH, or sun spots and revealing a fresher, healthier, and more radiant complexion.

Exfoliating Toners

Exfoliating toners are often a cocktail of acids (like AHAs, BHAs, and PHAs) and hydrating or conditioning agents. These ingredients all work together to buff away dead skin cells and regulate oil production while delivering replenishing and nourishing ingredients back into the skin. While exfoliating toners are capable of providing a healthy balance of hydration and treatment, this doesn't mean that it's okay to overuse them. When integrating exfoliating toners into your routine, be slow and steady, as they're still capable of stripping, irritating, or drying out your complexion.

One of the most common errors I see in skincare is over-exfoliating. With acne-prone skin, it's easy to feel desperate for results. So when something seems to be helping your skin, I understand that using it as much as possible feels like the wise thing to do. But as much as exfoliating is helpful, over-exfoliating, truthfully, can be the root cause of your acne flare-ups, dryness, and dullness. A good rule of thumb is to integrate an exfoliator into your routine once a week and, if your skin responds well, increase it to twice a week.

AM I OVER-EXFOLIATING?

Signs You're Over-Exfoliating Your Skin

Irritation   Redness   Dry patches   Breakouts

Chemical vs. Physical Exfoliators

I have my own biases when it comes to the chemical versus physical exfoliator debate. But ultimately the decision is dependent on what you are trying to improve when it comes to your skin and your specific concerns.

Physical exfoliators are products with grains or microbeads that—you guessed it—physically remove the dead skin from the surface of your face to reveal smoother, more radiant skin underneath. Generally speaking, people who don't suffer from consistent acne or pigmentation issues enjoy using a physical exfoliator, as the results are more about smoothing out the skin, rather than improving specific skin issues. The skincare community tends to regard the physical exfoliator as a kind of old-school formula due to its reputation for creating "microtears," microscopic tears in the skin caused by abrasion. If you're attached to using physical exfoliators, make sure you use very fine, gentle grains and that you don't apply excessive pressure onto the product as you apply it.

Chemical exfoliators use acids like AHAs, BHAs, and PHAs to encourage dead skin to slough off. Although modern-day shoppers have attached a negative connotation to the word *chemical* (we're accustomed to seeing "chemical free" on cleaning supplies and body lotions), when used carefully and sparingly, chemical exfoliators can actually be a much gentler option than physical exfoliators.

ESSENCES

Essences, also known as "beauty waters," are hydrating skincare products that were created and popularized in Japanese and Korean cosmetics. While many find the distinction between serums, moisturizers, toners, and essences to be confusing, the job of an essence is relatively simple: to deeply hydrate, condition, and replenish the skin. If moisturizer locks in hydration, essence is what ensures there is hydration present to lock in. Not all essences are the same—some are on the thinner, more watery side, while others are thicker and goopier—but they do all generally include moisturizing ingredients that promote a dewier, healthier, more nourished complexion. Essences are, of course, an incredibly helpful step for anyone with dry skin. But sensitive and/or mature skin types can also benefit from a daily essence, as they're typically formulated with replenishing and barrier-strengthening ingredients.

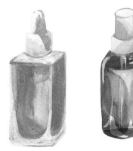

SERUMS AND AMPOULES

Serums and ampoules are typically regarded as the most daunting and mystifying part of the ten-step routine.

There are hundreds of different kinds of serums and ampoules, each one with a different texture and functionality. Although it can seem intimidating at first, becoming fluent in the art of serums and ampoules is *a lot* easier than you think. And once you understand their ways, you've conquered one of the most valuable treatment steps in the skincare game.

So, let's start with the basics: what's a serum and what's an ampoule? A serum is a lightweight, fast-absorbing, concentrated liquid that delivers active 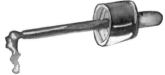 ingredients deep into the skin. Serums are used as a treatment step to satisfy your skin's specific needs, whether it be acne fighting, hydrating, or firming. Generally speaking, I use serums daily, in both my morning and evening routines: a vitamin C serum in my morning routine and a niacinamide serum in my evening routine.

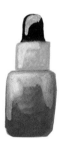 When I first learned about ampoules, I was told that they are a super-charged, doubly concentrated serum, kind of like a serum on steroids. Unlike serums, which are generally formulated for regular use, ampoules were initially created to be used for a limited amount of time, acting as a hyperintensive treatment. I was originally told by skincare lovers (both friends and editors alike) that you should use one every day for a few days *or* once every two weeks, less as an integral part of your routine and more as a skincare pick-me-up when you want to give your skin some supplementary TLC.

But these days, the serums versus ampoules debate is becoming less important—as if the skincare community woke up one day and realized the two terms were, more than anything, a way for brands to get us to buy more of the same stuff. So, what I'm saying is this: it's okay to group serums and ampoules together as one thing. There, I said it. There's really, at the end of the day, not that big of a difference between the two in terms of how they affect your skin.

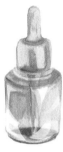

I don't believe in a set, one-size-fits-all approach when it comes to how often you should use your serums and ampoules. Pay attention to the ingredients (part two will help inform if there are things in your serum that should be used only in moderation) and then play around with them in your routine—if your skin looks a little greasy or you're breaking out, hold back. If your skin looks great using your serums and ampoules every day, that's okay too! Just listen to your skin and, as with any product, be sure to integrate them into your routine slowly.

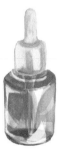

But wait, because there *is* one make-or-break rule when it comes to serums and ampoules: you can use as many serums and ampoules in your routine as you want (though I would personally cap it at two or three), as long as you're layering them from thinnest to thickest in consistency when you use them. Throwing on a bunch of serums willy-nilly without layering them in this particular way is actually a huge waste of money. Think about it: a thin, watery serum won't be able to penetrate past a thick, oily ampoule. It will just sit on

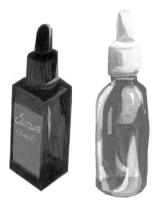

the surface of your skin. When you layer your products thinnest to thickest, your skin is able to properly absorb each product, maximizing its benefits.

Nine times out of ten, when someone tells me they don't think serums really do anything, it's because they're not subscribing to this small but mighty layering rule. Hand on heart—once you start noticing how the texture of your serums and ampoules affects the outcome of your skin, you won't be able to stop.

FACE MASKS

Face masks are an intensive skincare treatment that can help tend to a wide variety of concerns. As they typically require more time than your other skincare steps—around ten to fifteen minutes—they're usually intended to be used only once or twice a week, or as a kind of special indulgence.

There are tons of different kinds of masks available, but they can generally be separated into two categories: sheet and wash-off.

Sheet Masks

A sheet mask is a face-shaped fabric, usually made of fibers like cellulose or cotton, soaked in a potent essence liquid. Sheet masks work as an occlusive treatment, creating a physical barrier that prevents the evaporation of the ingredients while also encouraging the skin to absorb the essence. They should be applied in your nighttime skincare routine, either in lieu of your essence and serums or after them. All masks include directions for use, including how long to wear the mask. When your timer is up, remove the mask and pat the excess liquid into your skin. Sheet masks are suitable for all skin types (there are ones made specifically for oilier skin), but as they are drenched in a nourishing essence, they're especially good for dry or sensitive skin types.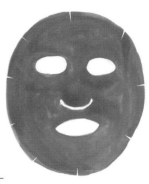

Wash-Off Masks

Unlike sheet masks, wash-off masks are formulated to be worn for a certain amount of time and then removed with lukewarm water. There are *tons* of wash-off masks on the market, but some of the most popular include clay-based

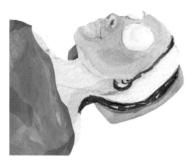

masks, charcoal-based masks, exfoliating masks, and hydrating masks. People tend to prefer a wash-off mask over a sheet mask given their ability to give a really deep clean to the pores. Not to mention, sheet masks are often single use, so wash-off masks are a more environmentally conscious option.

EYE CREAMS

The eye area is one of the most sensitive parts of the face—the skin is particularly thin and therefore more susceptible to dryness, fine lines, and wrinkles. Eye creams are treatments made specifically for the precious skin around the eyes and can help hydrate, plump, and rejuvenate the undereye area. A common misconception is that eye creams are a waste of money—that a moisturizer can work just as well at treating the undereye area. The truth is, overall facial moisturizers are not formulated with the undereye skin in mind, so they can actually clog or irritate that delicate area.

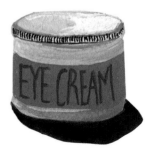

What About Dark Circles?

Dehydration is one of the biggest contributing factors to dark circles. Drinking lots of water and applying eye cream daily can help nourish and moisturize the area, which *may* help improve your dark circles. However, consistent dark circles are often the result of genetics (I can thank both my parents for mine!) making them particularly tricky to treat with topical creams. There's some evidence that suggests retinol-infused eye creams can help, but keeping your undereye area nice and hydrated, and occasionally reaching for a peachy-undertone concealer might be the most reliable way to tackle stubborn bags.

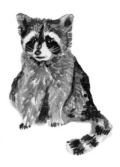

RETINOIDS

While retinoids are known to be some of the most effective skincare products available, there are some catches: your skin will possibly experience flaking, breakouts, redness, tightness, or irritation for an adjustment period of up to a month when you first start using them. And the truth of the matter is, even after your skin adapts, you probably won't see visible results for another six

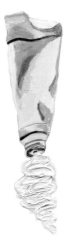

weeks. But with retinoids, there are major rewards for your patience: smoother, more radiant, and plumper skin.

Retinoids come in all different strengths and formulas. As I mentioned in part two, there are prescription retinoids that you can get from a dermatologist, and there are over-the-counter retinols that you can find in stores. Prescription retinoids are stronger, so, yes, the adjustment period will likely be more intense, but you'll see greater results sooner. Over-the-counter retinol isn't as strong, so while your purging period might not be as bad, the results will be milder.

How Should I Start Using a Retinoid?

When it comes to starting a retinoid, less is more. Start by applying a tiny, pea-sized amount of a formula with a lower concentration (0.01 percent if you're nervous and want to start *really* slow or 0.25 to 0.3 percent if you want a pretty low dosage with faster results) once a week and see how your skin responds. Over a few weeks, slowly up your usage to twice a week.

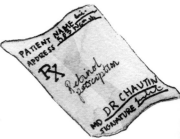

While prescription retinoids show faster, stronger results on the skin, it's common for first-time users to begin with low-concentration, over-the-counter retinols to acclimate their skin. That way, if they're looking for faster, more dramatic results later on, their skin will have built up a tolerance so they can then use a prescription retinoid like Retin-A. Regardless of your level of skin sensitivity, if you're using a retinoid in your skincare routine, you can benefit from the use of healing and hydrating ingredients on off days to prevent skin flare-ups.

Cream vs. Oil

While all prescription retinoids are cream based, over-the-counter retinol can come in a cream formula, blended in with your nighttime moisturizer, or in a more occlusive, oil-based formula. Oil-based formulas are better suited for people with drier or more sensitive skin types, while creams might be better for those with oilier skin types.

Where in Your Routine Should Retinoids Go?

This is a little tricky! When to apply your retinoid is all contingent on your skin type and the formula you're using. If you're using a prescription retinoid cream,

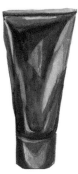

it can be applied before or after your moisturizer. Or, if you have very sensitive skin, it can also be sandwiched in between your moisturizer (moisturizer, retinoid, moisturizer). If you are using an over-the-counter retinol, it should be used either before your moisturizer or *as* your moisturizer if it's delivered in a night-cream formula.

MOISTURIZERS

No matter your skin type, moisturizers are excellent for helping your skin retain a healthy balance of hydration. Moisturizers have both preventative and treatment qualities: they lock in moisture while also ensuring that the skin doesn't get extremely dry again in the future. Moisturizers do this by holding water in the stratum corneum, the outermost layer of skin.

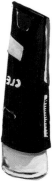

How to Choose a Moisturizer That's Right for You

There's a moisturizer for every skin type. If your skin is naturally very dry, itchy, or tight, thicker formulas that incorporate rich

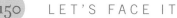

ingredients such as glycerin, shea butter, or ceramides will help nourish and condition the skin. If you're naturally oily and acne prone, thinner lotions or gels that use ingredients like hyaluronic acid and panthenol will moisturize the skin without being too thick or greasy.

Moisturizer vs. Face Oil

Face oils should be added to your skincare arsenal if you struggle with an unquenchable dryness (whether that be only in the winter or year-round) that a standard moisturizer just hasn't seemed to satisfy. Face oils are often (but not always) a blend of plant oils, which are wonderful sources of antioxidants and help replenish and protect the skin. Unlike moisturizers, popular face oils don't often incorporate intensive, hydration-boosting ingredients such as ceramides, peptides, and hyaluronic acid.

Face oil should be applied last, after your moisturizer, as it is a thicker consistency. In winter months, it can be useful to "seal in" your moisturizer at night with a layer of face oil, ensuring your skin absorbs it while you sleep.

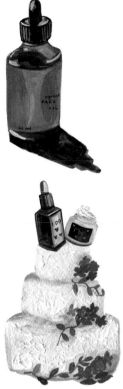

SLEEPING PACKS

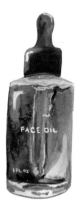

Sleeping packs may have a funny name, but they're essentially overnight masks that you apply as the final step in your evening skincare routine (in lieu of moisturizer and a face oil), which give you an extra boost of moisture and treatment. Depending on the formula, they can be a bit heavy for nightly use, but can be great as a weekly treatment (much like a regular face mask), before a special occasion, or when you want to deliver a big burst of hydration to your skin. Unlike a face mask, a sleeping pack doesn't need to be removed or washed off—just apply it and let it absorb.

I know what you're thinking: "Is this just a fancy way of saying moisturizer?" The truth is . . . kind of! But unlike your standard moisturizer that works to seal in all your other products, sleeping packs can make an ideal one-stop shop if you want a low-effort, one-step skincare routine without having to skip all your favorite ingredients. Some sleeping packs include power actives like retinol or lactic acid or

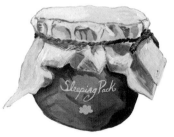

high concentrations of snail mucin or propolis that might be too sticky to wear during the daytime, but are perfect for waking up with glowy skin.

SUNSCREENS

Sunscreen is essential as the final step in your daytime skincare routine. It's not only the most powerful protectant against premature aging, it also protects the skin from harmful UV rays linked to skin cancer.

How to Choose a Sunscreen That's Right for You

It's important to select a sunscreen that provides your skin with maximum protection from harmful UV rays linked to premature aging and, more important, skin cancer. Your sunscreen should have broad-spectrum coverage to ensure that you're getting sufficient protection against both UVA and UVB rays from the sun. As we discussed in the previous part, there are a few types of sunscreens to choose from.

WHAT DOES THE SPF RATING MEAN?

SPF measures how well a sunscreen protects skin from skin-burning UVB rays. If a product has SPF 15, it means that the average tester got about fifteen times more UVB protection than they would have if they weren't wearing sunscreen. Most dermatologists advise using sunscreens with an SPF of at least 30 to 50.

BROAD-SPECTRUM COVERAGE

The sun doesn't produce exclusively UVB rays; it also emits UVA rays, which dermatologists have discovered are more closely linked to premature aging and skin cancers such as melanoma. The term "broad spectrum" refers to a product that is capable of protecting skin from both types of rays—UVA and UVB. To ensure sufficient protection, the FDA requires all products labeled as broad spectrum to take a "critical wavelength test" to prove the sunscreen adequately protects skin against UVA rays at 370 nanometers, as well as a supplementary test that ensures the UVB protection is over SPF 15. It's important that your sunscreen has broad-spectrum coverage to ensure that you're getting sufficient protection against both UVA and UVB rays from the sun.

What Is Blue Light?

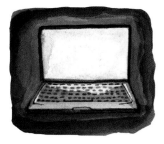

Blue light, also called HEV (high-energy visible) light, is different from UVB and UVA rays—it's a higher-energy, deeper-penetrating light that's part of the spectrum of visible light. While the primary source of blue light is the sun, research in recent years has shown that blue light can also come from phones and computers, proving to be another source of skin damage that can lead to premature aging, as well as redness, swelling, and hyperpigmentation.

While blue light from computers is something that has only been studied since 2010, more and more brands are introducing formulas that can protect the skin from HEV light, as well as UVA and UVB rays.

Sunscreen Application

The appropriate amount of sunscreen is about half a teaspoon for your face and neck, and about two tablespoons for your whole body. It's important to double check that you've gotten all those not-so-obvious places: Did you get your neck? Your ears? Your hands? The bridge of your nose?

SunScreen

MAKE SURE YOU DON'T MISS THIS!

EARS ✓

BACK OF NECK ✓

BRIDGE OF NOSE ✓

HANDS ✓

SUN
SPF 35

HOW TO APPLY PRODUCTS

While the physical method by which you apply products might seem like an afterthought, tactical application can actually help your products absorb and work better, while also ensuring that you're not damaging your skin.

There are a few different application methods: rubbing, patting, pianoing, and massaging. And while the best way to do it can vary from step to step, there are two rules of thumb:

1. Be gentle—being too rough or aggressive can trigger inflammation, irritation, or even premature aging.
2. Always move in upward motions—gravity is constantly trying to pull our skin downward, and we want to fight against that in order to have bouncy, lively skin.

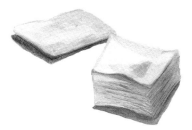

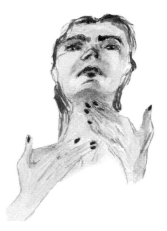

Rubbing

Cleansers are best applied by gently rubbing the product into the skin in circular motions, which can help dissolve makeup and stimulate blood flow. The rubbing motion can also help activate any sudsing agents that help the product clean better.

Patting

When it comes to toners, essences, serums, and moisturizers, it could be argued that they absorb better and are gentler on the skin when patted in. The patting motion encourages product immersion without tugging or yanking. Apply the product to your hands, then rub your two palms together; this will heat up the product and also evenly distribute it. Then, gently press it into the skin until you feel it sinking in.

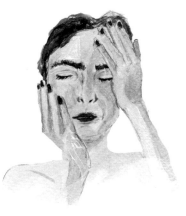

Pianoing

Yes, that's right—pianoing is when you apply products to your skin by gently tapping your fingers up and down your face until the product is adequately absorbed. Imagine your face is a piano keyboard and you're playing a lively song. Not only does this method allegedly stimulate and activate the muscles in the face (which helps with circulation), it also can be better than patting at encouraging thicker or stickier skincare to absorb into the skin. Also, since pianoing is particularly 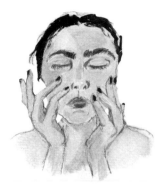 dainty and kind on the skin, it's a great way to apply products on particularly sensitive and tender areas of the face, like the undereye area!

FACIAL MASSAGING

Facial massaging is a treatment, often done with moisturizer or face oil, in which you *very gently* knead, rub, and massage your body's natural pressure points to decrease puffiness, improve circulation, and release tension in your face. You can get this treatment done during professional facials or do it at

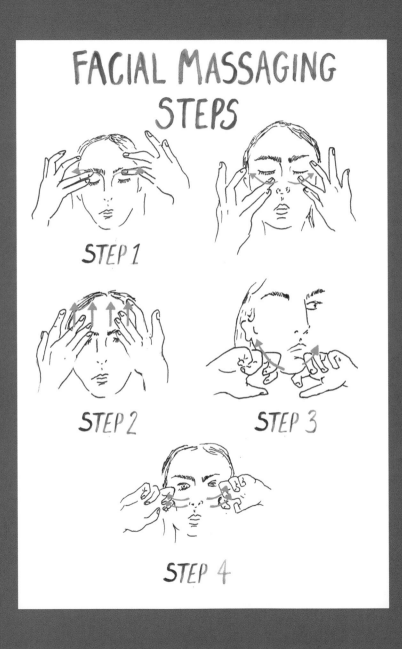

home with just your fingers. Depending on your skin type, it can be done anywhere from three times a week to once a month.

How to Facial Massage

Apply a moisturizer or face oil to your face to ensure your fingers glide easily over your skin.

STEP ONE: DEPUFF YOUR EYES
Using your ring fingers, gently press on the inner corner of your eyes (in between your eye and the side of your nose) and glide your fingers up, moving right underneath your eyebrows towards the outer tip of your brows, by your temples. Do this a few times. Then work the undereye area, starting again at the inner corner of your eyes and gently gliding down and over your undereye bags and then up towards the tip of your brows in a u-shape.

STEP TWO: SMOOTH YOUR FOREHEAD
Press your fingers in between your brows and, pressing down, glide them up towards your hairline. Repeat this across your forehead, working your way out, until you've massaged your entire forehead. Repeat as many times as you feel necessary.

 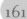

STEP THREE: DEFINE AND MASSAGE YOUR JAWLINE

Pinch your jawbone with your knuckles close to your chin. From your chin, glide them along your jawline up towards your ears.

STEP FOUR: LIFT YOUR CHEEKS

Pinch the apples of your cheeks with your knuckles, and then glide your knuckles, along the hollows of your cheeks, towards your ears.

What About This Jade Roller or Gua Sha Tool I Bought?

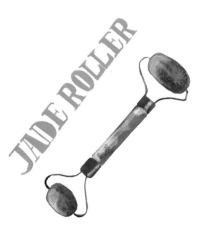

The above facial treatment can also be achieved with a gua sha or jade roller tool, which brands *claim* can more acutely target hard-to-reach pressure points on the skin. While I think using hands works just as well, the major benefit of these tools is that they can be stored in the fridge. Using a cold tool to massage your face adds extra de-puffing and de-swelling benefits.

Throughout this part, we've explored all the different avenues of skincare—the variations of cleansers, toners, exfoliators, and essences—and learned what they are capable of doing for your skin. In the next part, you're going to take what you've learned and fit it to your schedule, so you can carefully and thoughtfully build a routine that makes sense for you. It would be completely unrealistic to expect that everyone is capable of doing a double-digit-long skincare routine every day—in fact, it sometimes feels like a small miracle when we even get up and wash our face, and that's okay! Throughout part four of this book, we're going to talk about how this all pertains to you: how you can create a routine that's enough to help you achieve your optimal skin health, with a number of steps that you'll realistically find time for every day, whether that's two, five, or eight!

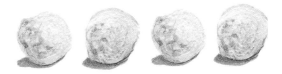

PART FOUR

Building a Routine

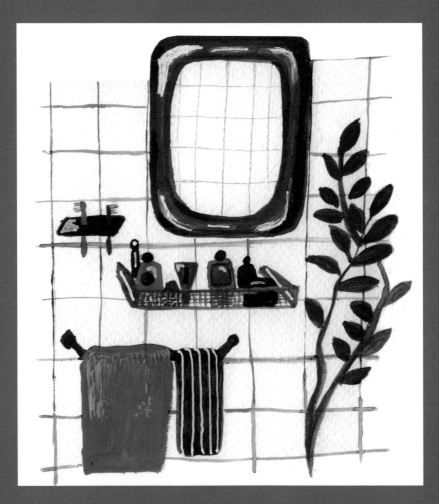

When thinking about products, it's important to take your daily life into consideration: Do you tend to wash your face before dinner, or do you do it right before you pass out? Do you skip steps already? In skincare, consistency is key—on average, it takes a whole thirty days to gauge what a product is doing for your skin. So, if you know you're short on time in the mornings and evenings, creating a giant routine that you know you won't end up doing will just set yourself up for failure. And there's no shame in smaller routines! Simple routines are truly just as effective—it's just important that the products you are using are right for your skin type.

Equally, maximalist routines can be wonderfully nurturing. Don't get me wrong: there are certainly areas where you can overdo skincare (we see this most with over-exfoliation), but treating your skin to layers of deeply nourishing and replenishing ingredients can be great. Your dedication to pampering your skin can be particularly important in winter, when your skin is most susceptible to irritation or dehydration. It's also important to give your skin extra love when you are using intensive treatments such as retinoids,

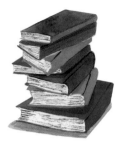

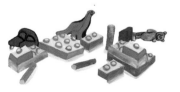

which can often trigger extreme sensitivity and require an equal balance of moisturizing and soothing properties.

Something I frequently hear from people, most often those with extremely busy jobs or kids, is that they'd really love to take the time to create a healthy skincare routine for themselves but fear that they won't be able to keep up with the daily maintenance. In this day and age, it's easy to be overwhelmed by the constant influx of information thrown at us and the high standards we're consistently held to. Socially, we're expected to stay up-to-date on the buzzy TV shows, books, and films so that we can participate in conversations with colleagues and friends. Plus, we're told to work out three times a week by studies in magazines or the news, not to mention most of our time is spent working. So, the idea of a skincare routine—carving out time to pamper yourself with toners and creams and serums—can feel like yet another task to add to your ever-growing to-do list.

But unlike other aspects of your life, which often move at a rapid, unforgiving, unwavering speed, a skincare routine is entirely adaptable to your needs and schedule. A skincare routine, at its core, should feel self-nurturing and meditative. No one else but you is in charge of it. How many steps you have

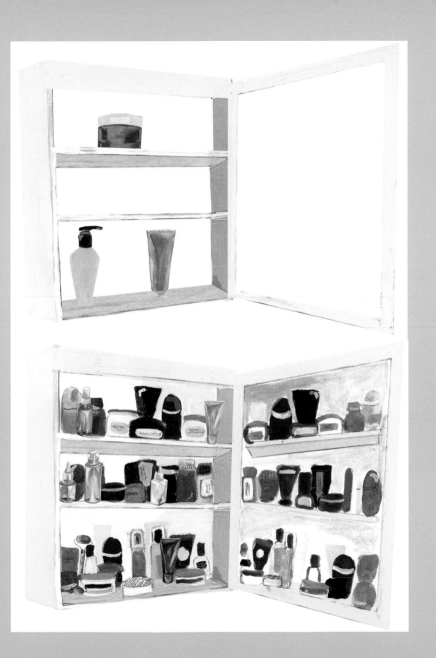

time for, what you want to use, what you think will help—all of it is your choice. If you only have time for one step today, that's okay. If you have time for four, that's great too. It's all about executing what you can based on the time you've allotted yourself, what your skin needs, and, really, what feels *nice* to do. When I meet someone new, often they'll say something along the lines of "You'd be ashamed of how little I do to my skin." But, honestly, if a minimal, concise routine works for your skin and schedule, I support it. As long as you're using sun protection!

As we discussed in the previous part, there's no point in rushing out to buy products to fill a lengthy ten-step routine if you know you're not going to stick to it. Personally, I like to keep my morning routine pretty quick and easy, with just the necessities, because I know I'm naturally not an early riser and am always running a bit late. For me, that means cleansing (situationally—sometimes I don't if I feel I haven't sweat in my sleep), vitamin C for helping fade any hyperpigmentation, which is a consistent issue for me, moisturizer, and SPF.

In the evenings, however, I like to be more indulgent. I find my skincare routine to be a relaxing and genuinely therapeutic practice, helping me "turn

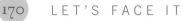

off" from the day and wind down for the evening. I double cleanse, sometimes exfoliate, pat in an essence, and then lock it in with a moisturizer and face oil. Five-ish steps, for me, is the right number—the one that I know I'll stick to every evening, no matter how tired, grumpy, or perhaps even tipsy I might be. Certainly, there are lazy Sundays where I might throw in a sheet mask here or there, but for the most part that five-step, fifteen-minute routine is what I stick to.

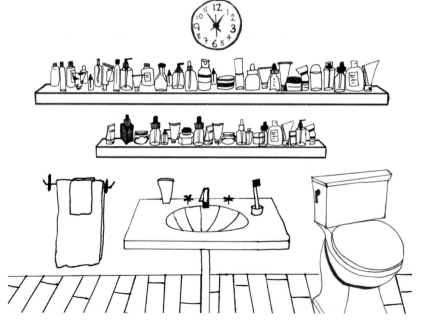

STARTING A ROUTINE FROM SCRATCH

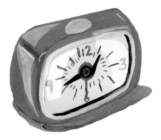

When initially curating a routine from scratch, patience is vital to ensuring maximum effectiveness. In order to identify the results of a product, new skincare should be integrated into your regimen slowly, one product at a time. Overzealousness can be your worst enemy when it comes to skincare: excitedly trying four new products at once can make it especially hard to identify what's doing what for your skin. Trust me, it's easier to be conservative with your product integration initially than to try and backtrack later.

Generally speaking, a product should also be used for at least a month before you can make a positive claim about its effectiveness (I tend to know earlier if my skin just *hates* something). Your skin cells regenerate every thirty days, so that window of time makes for a good rule of thumb to see how your skin interacts with a product throughout a full cycle. Of course, there are exceptions to this rule—moisturizers, for example, show results more quickly, pretty much instantly after you start using a new one, while retinoids take about six months to reveal their maximum potential.

How to Tell If a Product Isn't Working

Sometimes, products do more than just not show results—they can make your skin worse, causing irritation, additional breakouts, or even an allergic reaction. If you start seeing the signs of an adverse reaction, stop using the product immediately. I like to keep track of products that cause my skin to react poorly, since comparing the ingredients in products my skin hasn't liked helps me identify whether a particular ingredient is to blame.

Signs of a Bad Reaction

Irritation

Dryness

Tenderness

Flakiness

Redness

Breakouts in unusual areas

Retinoids are an exception to this rule, as purging
   or flakiness is often a sign that they're working.

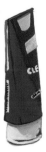

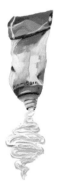

The three essentials of skincare are your cleanser, moisturizer, and sunscreen. These three steps give your skin what it needs on a most basic level: purifying the skin of dirt, locking in moisture, and protecting it from harsh ultraviolet rays. While these three steps are the backbone of any routine, they don't often provide the skin with a lot of active treatment—they can keep your skin happy, but you won't see much overwhelming *improvement* if you have a specific issue you're hoping to target. If you suffer from pigmentation, textural issues, or acne, most treatment will come from your exfoliator or retinoid. Exfoliators and retinoids are the workhorses of any skincare routine. You can still have a good regimen without them, but if you are really trying to change something about your skin (whether it be persistent acne or deep wrinkles), these are the steps you should consider. They intensely resurface, heal, and add radiance to the skin, and they are often where you see the most dramatic results.

As exfoliators are capable of such results, it's important to introduce them in isolation and be patient, applying them steadily once or twice

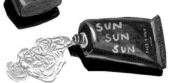

a week for thirty days before integrating any other new products. With this method, you can gauge the positive or negative effects the exfoliator is having on your skin, so you can make a more informed decision about how often you should use it and what else your skin needs, if anything.

Retinoids, on the other hand, are a slower burn and can take about six months to reveal their full potential on your skin. The first month of using a retinoid can be frustrating—as your skin adjusts to the intense formula, it's common to see side effects such as flakiness, redness, tenderness, and breakouts. However, retinoids can have some of the most powerful results in skincare: they help get rid of old skin cells and push up young, fresh skin that's more luminous, tighter, and clearer.

As we talked about in part two, retinoids and exfoliators should never be used together in the same routine. Both are extremely powerful resurfacing products; together, they can severely irritate the skin. To use both safely, some people like to alternate between a month with retinoids and a month with exfoliators. If you're deciding between the two, I would recommend starting out with an exfoliator, as they are less of a commitment than retinoids.

Both exfoliators and retinoids are capable of stripping the skin (though retinoids are more aggressively so at first), which means they work well when paired with an essence, which acts as a kind of soothing, calming surge of hydration into the skin. This can help replenish the moisture that your exfoliator or retinoid has potentially stripped it of. While essences are typically moisture supplements, rather than active treatments, I still believe they should be used for thirty days, with no other serums or ampoules, to see how effective the product is on your skin. Vitamin C serums are another product that can reveal huge results, but only if used consistently for at least thirty days.

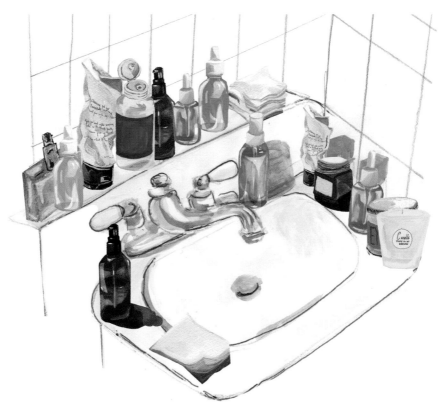

EDITING A SKINCARE ROUTINE

Much like building your routine, editing or paring it down should be done thoughtfully and methodically. Removing products all at once can create a shock to your skin, especially if you have been using the same products for an extended period of time. A slow removal process—cutting or replacing products one by one—will allow you to assess the necessity of the products you already use. For example, if you take out your exfoliator and start breaking out, you know that your skin really likes an ingredient in that product. Same goes for swapping in new products; you can easily connect a positive or negative reaction to the one that's new.

SKINCARE AS "YOU TIME"

Instead of thinking of it as burdensome, try and think of your skincare routine as an opportunity to check in with yourself twice a day. It's a time to unpack your experiences, plan for upcoming events, and allow your aspirations, anxieties, and goals to rise to the surface. I find using this time to prepare for big meetings or interviews especially helpful. Sometimes I speak to myself out loud as I do my skincare routine: I give myself affirmations, or, if I'm anxious for an event, I practice what I'm going to say. Before public speaking, big meetings, or interviews, I tend to get incredibly nervous—not only do I privately suffer (an aggressively bubbling stomach, racing heart, and shortness of breath are all the norm), but my shaky hands and voice are a quick giveaway to anyone I'm speaking to. Rehearsing hypothetical answers or scenarios in the privacy of my own bathroom, completely by myself, helps me feel more confident in myself and my words, which takes the edge off my nerves. Truth be told, if I didn't have a skincare routine, I'm not sure I would carve out the time to execute this kind of preparation, but I know it's the key to my success in otherwise anxiety-producing settings.

I find the choice to complete my skincare routine an impressive act of self-determination—it's symbolic of me starting or ending my day at its fullest potential. I'm making the choice to prioritize taking care of myself.

Of course, a skincare routine isn't a singular solution to any mental health issues, but it is an opportunity to take more time alone with yourself. I like to think of it as a standing, twice-a-day date to check in with yourself and where you're at.

Equally, a skincare routine should never feel like a product of anyone else's expectations. No one but you should be the guiding force in your decision to

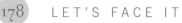

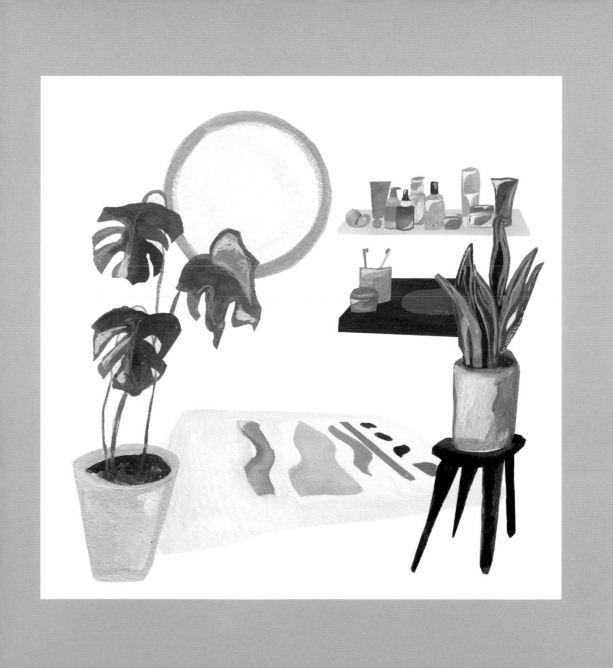

build a routine. As someone who has struggled with fluctuating acne my whole life, I understand the painful and often nuanced emotions one can experience when looking in a bathroom mirror. I used to feel like I couldn't even look at myself, so how could anyone else? I also sympathize with the increased stakes at play for acne sufferers who obsessively try and test new products; so many times, I've applied products out of sheer desperation, hoping that an improvement in my skin could somehow repair my confidence. The most important thing to remember in these kinds of situations is that building a healthy relationship with your skin is a process that takes time. No matter how well you understand the ins and outs of skincare—the research you do into the newest and most innovative products, the blogs you read—reaching a place of long-term acceptance with your skin doesn't happen overnight. Certain products may have the ability to improve and heal skin issues, but it's up to you to create a healthy environment for your skin to continue to flourish—without picking, overanalyzing, or scrutinizing. Unlearning the things you've taught yourself about your skin and creating boundaries with yourself—in my case this meant actually removing my bathroom mirror for a period of time—is necessary for the continuous improvement of your relationship with your skin.

From a young age, I was enamored of my mother's diligent beauty routine. Each morning before taking me to school, she would massage creams into her skin, run patchouli-scented oils through the ends of her hair, and swipe a teal kohl eyeliner along her eyelids. I was fascinated by the transformative nature of this routine—less so in the literal, physical sense and more so in how it was able to completely shift her state of mind. There was Mom before the bathroom, and there was Mom after it. She would stumble in lethargic and grumpy but would emerge focused, energized, and ready to take on the day. In a Clark Kent–ish fashion, the woman who walked out of the

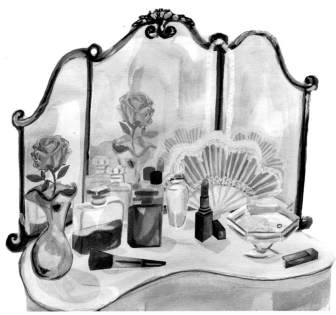

bathroom represented a super-charged version of the woman who entered it. It would take me until my early twenties, when I developed my own morning beauty routine, to realize that what she was experiencing were the self-motivating, revitalizing effects of prioritizing spending time with herself.

Despite the transformative benefits of skincare, I so often hear from people who struggle with making time for themselves in the middle of a busy day. Here are my tips and tricks for making time for your skincare routine:

1. Leave the party when you feel like it.

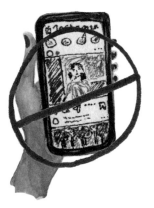

It's okay to feel antisocial, but I do want to let you know you've been checking your phone every three minutes. Let me guess: you want to go home, but you think if you leave now everyone will talk about what a weird mood you were in tonight. And now that I mention it, doesn't washing your face, getting in bed, and watching three episodes of TV sound just so utterly delightful? Set yourself free!

2. Stop looking at Instagram.

It's nine p.m. and you've been going down a toxic wormhole on Instagram for thirty minutes straight. It's okay, I'm not judging—we've all been there. When you come home from work or a long day, it can be nice to want to feel connected to friends by looking at Instagram or Twitter—this is a totally nor-

mal response to feeling isolated or overworked by a job. But it's just as important to use your precious free time to build and nurture that connection with
yourself. I know throwing on a sheet mask might not necessarily feel like the
most physically or mentally beneficial thing for your health. And, to a certain extent, that's true: a workout class or therapy will probably have greater,
longer-lasting effects on your health. But a sheet mask and the act of doing
your skincare is symbolic of something greater. It's a choice to do something
entirely for yourself.

3. Wake up fifteen minutes earlier.

If you're already an early riser, this advice
is likely something that's already in-
grained in your day-to-day schedule. But if, like me, you're the
type of person to risk your
whole career just to get an extra
ten or fifteen minutes of sleep,
let's talk. Previously, my skincare routines in the morning

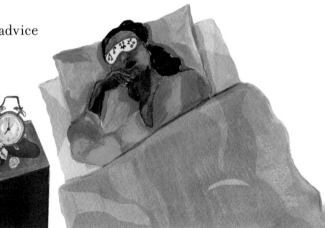

consisted of whatever time allowed: just slapping sunscreen on my face and bolting out the door. And while there's nothing wrong with this—I echo my previous statement about skincare routines being what makes sense for you and your schedule—waking up earlier has significantly improved my entire morning practice, and not just the time I spend on my skincare routine. Now, I wake up and make a pot of coffee, eat breakfast (something previously unheard of), and joyfully do my skincare routine. Sometimes, I'll even throw on a sheet mask while I read my *New York Times* Morning Briefing. Admittedly, this in large part has to do with the fact that my cat screams in my ear to wake me up in the morning, and I don't think, truly, I'll ever be the kind of person who wakes up at six a.m. by choice. Having said that, there are only twenty-four hours in the day. And if you're someone who works standard office hours and feels frustrated by how little time you have for yourself throughout the day, carving out extra time for yourself to do what makes you feel happy in the mornings can make a big difference.

SKIN PICKING

We've all looked in the mirror and felt that insatiable urge to start extracting any little bumps or spots we might see or feel on our skin. Have you noticed that once you begin, it's nearly impossible to actually stop yourself? There have been countless times I've gone to town on my skin, starting with a single blackhead and quickly escalating into a full attack on just about anything I could squeeze.

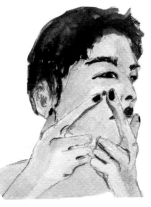

Now, more than ever, skin picking is being studied and observed as both a legitimate form of self-harm and a psychological compulsion. Skin picking is often a response to anxiety and stress, but it can also be a compulsion we partake in simply out of boredom or habit.

Stopping the habit of picking is actually more difficult than you would think. What's known to be the most effective way to deal with it is to rid your home of any tools and make small changes that make your environment less conducive to picking.

Ways to Stop Yourself from Picking

GETTING RID OF HARSH BATHROOM LIGHTS

Harsh lights that present an unrealistic perception of what you look like—a fluorescent, intensified version of your skin—can make even the smallest blackhead seem noticeable. Changing the bulbs in your bathroom to softer lighting is a great way to abate that harshness. When it comes to skin picking, the less you can see, the better.

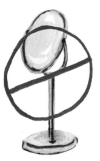

GETTING RID OF MAGNIFYING MIRRORS

Throw these out immediately. There is absolutely no need for anyone to have a magnifying mirror.

USING PIMPLE PATCHES

Out of sight, out of mind! Pimple patches are hydrocolloid patches that, when applied to a zit, help absorb excess oil, dirt, and bacteria. When you feel the urge to pick or extract a spot, throw a pimple patch on it.

ICING INSTEAD OF PICKING

This will give you the satisfaction of doing something pro-active, without the violence of picking your skin. Putting an ice cube wrapped in a cloth (or even a cold spoon) on the affected area will reduce some of the inflammation, pro-viding a similarly satisfying result.

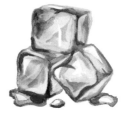

LIMITING YOUR TIME IN FRONT OF THE MIRROR

Ask a roommate, family member, or friend to time you (or just keep a casual eye on the clock) each time you go in the bathroom to wash your face.

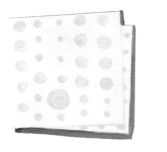

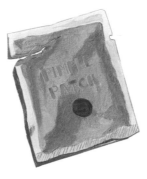

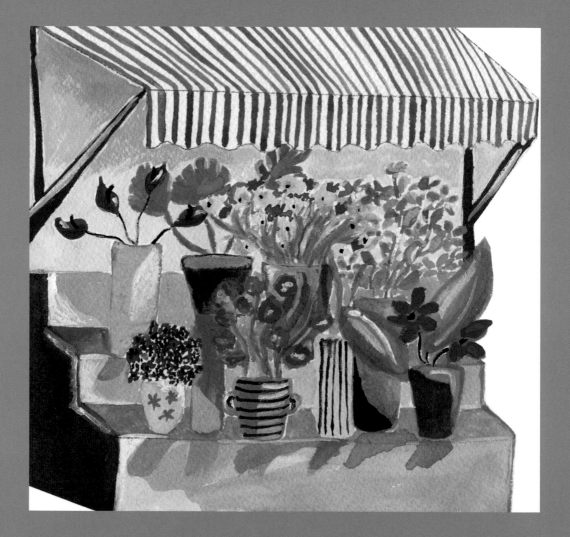

ON YOUR OWN

The appearance of busyness and being overworked have become symbols of success in our culture. We're conditioned to admire those who are so hard-working they barely have time to do anything for themselves. This celebration of stress makes us feel guilty when we prioritize our needs; we all feel like we aren't doing enough.

It's hard to rewire your brain to give yourself permission to indulge in things that just feel good. I'm constantly haunted by the idea that there's something else, something more productive I should be doing. For me, creating a skincare routine was my first step in ensuring I carve out more time for myself. The fifteen minutes I spend alone with myself in the mornings and evenings quickly became some of my most cherished moments—I feel intuitive, calm, and content.

But not all skincare routines are created equal. At the end of the day, your routine is an extension of yourself and your body. Throughout the course of this book, I've given you all the tools necessary for you to create a bespoke routine catered to you, your needs, and your schedule, however specific they might be. The five pillars of skincare are a guidebook you can constantly

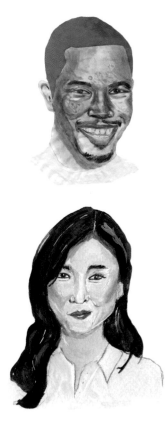

refer back to; they're your safety net that will steer you towards ingredients and products that make sense for you. Whether you're overwhelmed at a Sephora or wake up with a cluster of mystery spots all over your face, this book and the pillars of skincare will be here to re-center you. We're your rock, reminding you that your skin and the products you put on it are your friends, not your foes. Your skin is the largest organ of your body, and, because of that, it is often the loudest: it gets red when it's irritated, glowy when it's balanced, and tight when it's in need of moisture. It's a window into your body—your hormones, your sleep schedule, and your hydration levels. So don't freak out, because now's the time to listen to it.

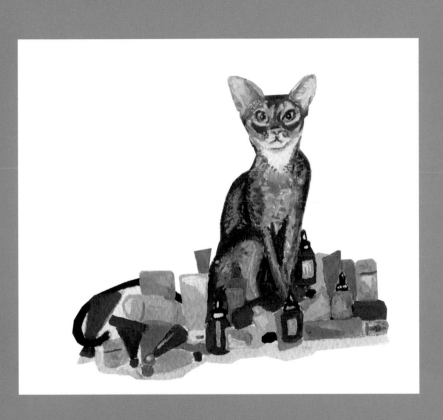

I would like to thank the many people
who made this book possible.

To my loyal support system—
Mom, Dad, Harley, Dean, Dom, and Jackson.
Thank you for believing in me.
I love you all so much.

To Dr. Loretta, Allison, Nicky, Laura, and Sofie—
thank you for your wisdom and patience with me.
I'm grateful for every second we spent putting
this book together.

Voracious / Little, Brown and Company
Hachette Book Group
1290 Avenue of the Americas, New York, NY 10104
littlebrown.com

First Edition: March 2021

Voracious is an imprint of Little, Brown and Company, a division of Hachette Book Group, Inc.
The Voracious name and logo are trademarks of Hachette Book Group, Inc.

The publisher is not responsible for websites (or their content) that are not owned
by the publisher.

The Hachette Speakers Bureau provides a wide range of authors for speaking events.
To find out more, go to hachettespeakersbureau.com or call (866) 376-6591.

Design by Bonni Leon-Berman
Illustrations by Laura Chautin

ISBN 978-0-316-54013-1
LCCN 2020942219

10 9 8 7 6 5 4 3 2 1

APS

Printed in China